Paediatric First Aid

CONTENTS

Paediatric First Aid is published by:
Instructuk Resources Ltd

Paediatric First Aid | ISBN 978-1-908597-04-5
8th Edition December 2019-12-01 : Printed December 2019

ROLE OF THE PAEDIATRIC FIRST AIDER

WHAT IS PAEDIATRIC FIRST AID?

In all of our lives, whether at work, home or at play, it is essential that we all know how to assist a child or infant who is sick, or has been injured.

Paediatric First Aid, as the term implies, is the initial treatment given to a child or infant who is injured or sick, prior to professional medical assistance arriving and taking over from you.

By reading this manual, it will not make you a doctor, paramedic or nurse, but by applying common sense and some basic life support skills, as well as providing care and confidence in your treatment for the casualty, you will learn skills that will enhance their well-being and in some very serious cases, possibly save their life.

Your prompt, safe and effective treatment could make a difference between life and death.

As a Paediatric First Aider, your priorities for the casualty fall into the following categories:

PRESERVE life
ALLEVIATE suffering
PREVENT the condition from worsening
PROMOTE recovery

For instance, if your casualty is suffering major blood loss as a result of a serious cut, then you can **preserve life** by offering treatment immediately and not waiting for professional help to sort it out for you. If you do nothing, then your casualty could bleed to death.

We can **alleviate suffering** by making the casualty more comfortable, reducing their pain levels and offering lots of care and attention.

We can **prevent further illness or injury** by applying a secure sterile dressing on the injured part in order to control the blood loss and prevent the risk of infection.

We can **promote recovery** by treating the casualty for shock and ringing for an ambulance.

DEFINITION OF PAEDIATRIC

The term paediatric refers to children and infants (babies). A child is deemed as being aged from 1 to the onset of puberty and an infant or baby, being aged under 1 year old.

If you are in any doubt on whether a child has reached the onset of puberty, then treat them as an adult, as little harm will come to them by adopting the adult protocols.

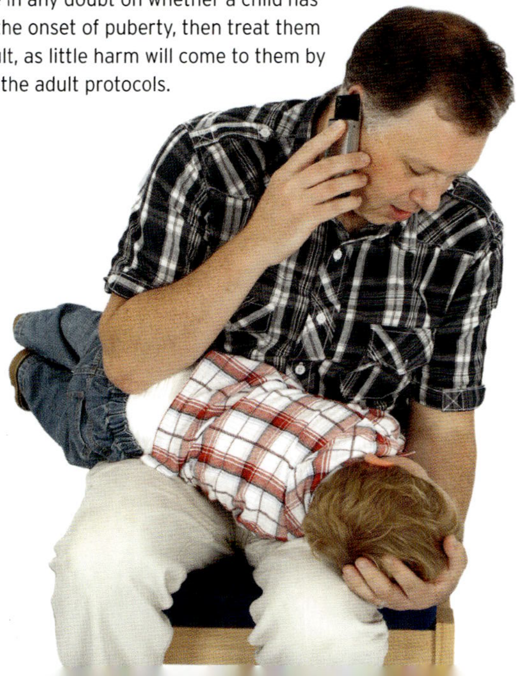

ACTS AND REGULATIONS

For some, you may have a responsibility in the workplace for First Aid. Should this be the case then you must be aware of legislation that ensures employers provide a duty of care, along with a First Aid provision for their employees, as well as non-employees and contractors visiting their premises.

THE HEALTH AND SAFETY AT WORK ACT 1974

This Act, also abbreviated to HSWA , HASWA or HASAWA , is an Act of the Parliament of the United Kingdom that currently defines the fundamental structure and authority for the encouragement, regulation and enforcement of workplace health, safety and welfare within the United Kingdom.

The Act defines general duties on employers, employees, contractors, suppliers of goods and substances for use at work, persons in control of work premises, and those who manage and maintain them, and persons in general.

THE MANAGEMENT OF THE HEALTH AND SAFETY AT WORK REGULATIONS 1999

These Regulations generally make more explicit what employers are required to do to manage health and safety under the Health and Safety at Work Act. Like the Act, they apply to every work activity, including the provision of First Aid. The main requirement for employers is to carry out a risk assessment. Employers with five or more employees need to record the significant findings of the risk assessment. Risk assessment should be straightforward in a simple workplace such as a typical office.

THE HEALTH AND SAFETY (FIRST AID) REGULATIONS 1981 (1982 IN NORTHERN IRELAND)

The Health and Safety (First-Aid) Regulations 1981 require employers to provide adequate and appropriate equipment, facilities and personnel to ensure their employees receive immediate attention if they are injured or taken ill at work.

PAEDIATRIC FIRST AID PROVISION

You should liaise with management and other First Aider's to ensure:

- **There is an adequate number of Paediatric First Aider's, First Aider's and Emergency First Aider's in place**
- **Appropriate equipment, kits and facilities are available**
- **A system is in place for incident and accident reporting**

It is vital that a risk assessment of First Aid needs is conducted to ensure that the correct level of provision is made.

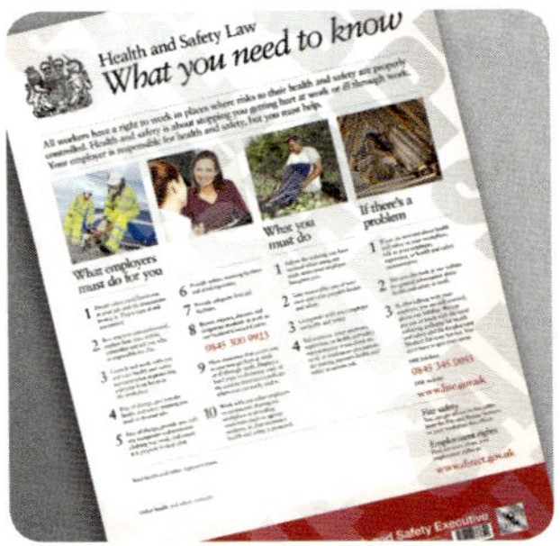

Where the risk assessment identifies the need for people to be available for rendering First Aid, then the employer should ensure that they are provided in sufficient numbers and at appropriate locations to enable First Aid to be administered without delay, should the occasion arise.

New guidance on the Regulations for employers was introduced in October 2013 (L74 - Third edition).

The following table will guide you in ensuring that you have sufficient numbers of trained First Aid personnel at your place of work.

1. From your risk assessment, what degree of hazard is associated with your work activities	2. How many employees do you have?	3. What First Aid personnel do you need?	4. What injuries and illnesses have previously occurred in your workplace	5. Have you taken account of the factors below that may affect your First Aid provision?
Low-hazard eg offices, shops, libraries	Fewer than 25	At least **1 appointed person**	• Ensure any injuries or illness that may occur can be dealt with by the First Aider's you provide • Where First Aider's are shown to be unnecessary, there is still a possibility of an accident or sudden illness, so you may wish to consider providing qualified First Aider's	• Inexperienced workers or employees with disabilities or particular health problems • Employees who travel a lot, work remotely or work alone • Employees who work out-of-hours • Premises spread out across buildings/floors • Workplace remote from the emergency services • Employees working at sites occupied by other employers • Planned & unplanned absences of first-aider/ appointed person • Members of the public who visit the workplace
	25 - 50	At least **1 EFAW** trained First Aider		
	More than 50	At least **1 FAW** trained First Aider for every 100 employed (or part thereof)		
Higher hazard eg light engineering and assembly work, food processing, warehousing, extensive work with dangerous machinery or sharp instruments, construction, chemical manufacture	Fewer than 5	At least **1 appointed person**		
	5 - 50	At least **1 EFAW** or **FAW** trained First Aider, depending on the type of injuries that may occur		
	More than 50	At least **1 FAW** trained First Aider for every 50 employed (or part thereof)		

Information supplied by Health & Safety Executive. The Health and Safety (First-Aid) Regulations 1981 L74 (Third edition 2013)

FIRST AID CONTAINERS

The minimum level of First Aid equipment is a suitably stocked and properly identified First Aid container.

Every employer should provide, for each work site, at least one First Aid container supplied with a sufficient quantity of First Aid materials suitable for the particular circumstances.

There is no mandatory list of items to be included in a First Aid container. The decision on what to provide, will be influenced by the findings of the First Aid needs assessment. As a guide, where work activities involve low hazards, a minimum stock of First Aid items might be:

- **A guidance leaflet**
- **20 individually wrapped plasters**
  (Assorted sizes)
- **2 sterile eye pads**
- **2 triangular bandages**
  (Individually wrapped and preferably sterile)
- **6 medium sterile wound dressings**
  (Individually wrapped and un-medicated)
- **2 large sterile wound dressings**
  (Individually wrapped and un-medicated)
- **At least 3 pairs of disposable gloves**
- **6 safety pins**

This is a suggested contents list only.

The contents of First Aid containers should be examined frequently and restocked soon after use. Sufficient supplies should be held in stock on site. Care should be taken to dispose of items safely once they reach their expiry date.

ADDITIONAL FIRST AID MATERIALS AND EQUIPMENT

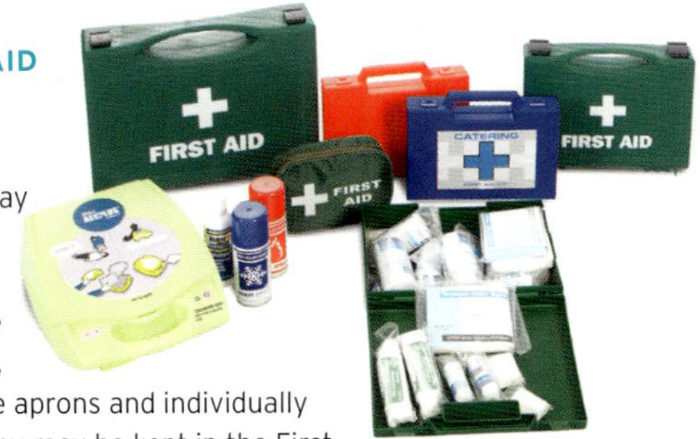

The needs assessment may indicate that additional materials and equipment are required, for example scissors, burns dressings, adhesive tape, disposable aprons and individually wrapped moist wipes. They may be kept in the First Aid container if there is room, or stored separately.

If mains tap water is not readily available for eye irrigation, at least a litre of sterile water or sterile normal saline (0.9%) in sealed, disposable containers should be provided. Once the seal has been broken, containers should not be kept for re-use. Containers should not be used beyond their expiry date.

First Aid at Work does not include giving tablets or medicines to treat illness.

The view of the Health and Safety Executive (HSE), is that the administration of medication by a First Aider is not part of a First Aid at Work training course, but you can assist an individual in taking it, if it is their own medication.

It is recommended that tablets and medicines should not be kept in the First Aid container.

However, the one exception is heart attacks. Therefore, for heart attack management, the First Aider must be able to assist a casualty in taking 150 – 300 mg of chewable aspirin and to advise them to chew it rather than swallow it whole, providing you are confident that the casualty is not allergic to it. If you are in any doubt, then you **MUST NOT** administer it. Aspirin **MUST NOT** be administered to anyone under the age of 16.

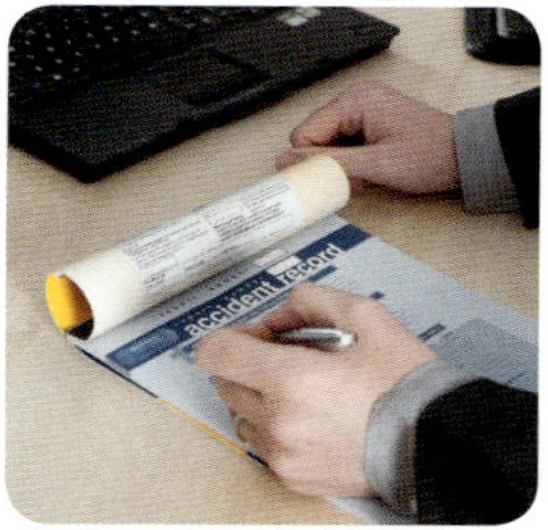

ACCIDENT AND INCIDENT REPORTING

Irrespective of the severity of the accident or incident, it is vital that all such occurrences be reported and filed by the employer.

Anyone can complete the accident book, and this book must comply with Data Protection legislation.

The accident book should be used as a useful reference for the purpose of ensuring that, where reasonably practicable, the same incident can be prevented from happening again.

An accident book can be purchased at most good book shops, or online from many First Aid supply shops.

The information that should be recorded includes:

- **The date, time and place of the incident**
- **Name and job of the injured or ill person**
- **Details of the injury/illness and what First Aid was given**
- **What happened to the casualty immediately afterwards?** (e.g. went back to work, went home, went to hospital)
- **Name and signature of the person reporting the incident**
- **The information must be kept in accordance with the Data Protection Act 2018**

Where the incident is of a severe nature, then the employer must comply with RIDDOR 2013.

RIDDOR is the law that requires employers, and other people in control of work premises, to report and keep records of:

- **Work-related accidents which cause death**
- **Work-related accidents which cause certain serious injuries (reportable injuries)**
- **Diagnosed cases of certain industrial diseases**
- **Certain 'dangerous occurrences' (incidents with the potential to cause harm)**

There are also special requirements for gas incidents.

Reporting certain incidents is a legal requirement. The report informs the enforcing authorities (HSE, local authorities and the Office for Rail Regulation (ORR)) about deaths, injuries, occupational diseases and dangerous occurrences, so they can identify where and how risks arise, and whether they need to be investigated.

Please visit **www.hse.gov.uk/riddor/** for full details of what is reportable.

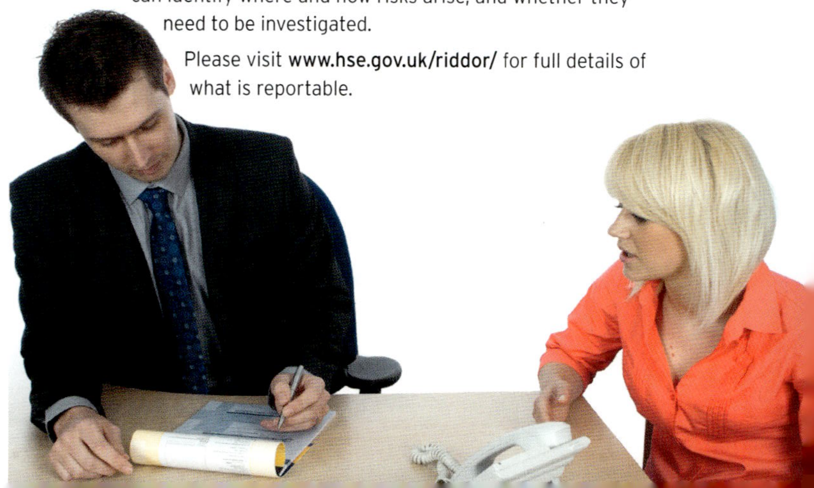

RESPONSIBILITIES

A paediatric First Aider has a number of responsibilities when dealing with an incident.

It is paramount that the incident is dealt with confidently and safely. The safety for all is important, including you, the casualty and any bystanders.

You must manage the incident and take control of the situation until professional medical help arrives and takes over. A bystander can be a great benefit to you, particularly if they are qualified in First Aid, so don't be afraid to summon help.

A bystander can make a telephone call, get a First Aid kit, return with the defibrillator if you have one, manage the crowd and traffic, and generally support you.

Your responsibilities can be broken up into the following categories:

- **Arrival at the scene**
- **Dealing with casualties**
- **Casualty communication**
- **Contacting the emergency services**
- **Prioritise the First Aid treatment**
- **Clearing up process and infection control**

ARRIVAL AT THE SCENE

Make the area safe and gather as much information about the incident as you can. The history of the incident and any casualty information about their illness or injury could help you decide your course of initial treatment.

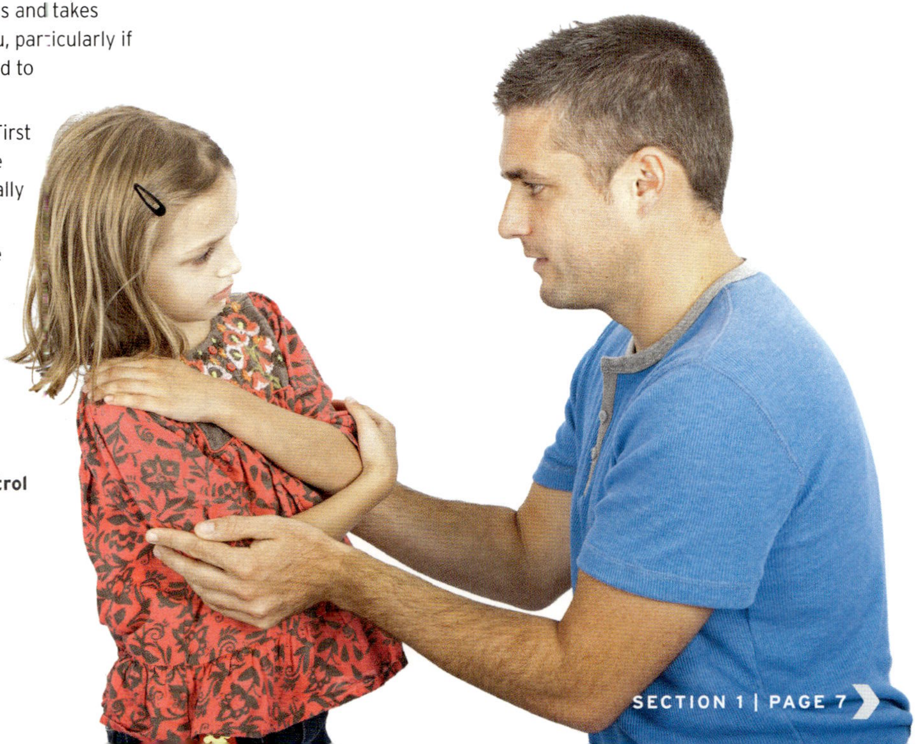

ROLE OF THE PAEDIATRIC FIRST AIDER continued

Ensure you have help at hand.

You are almost certain to be feeling nervous and anxious yourself, but be as confident as you can, and take control of the situation.

DEALING WITH CASUALTIES

- **Prioritise your treatment, particularly if you have multiple casualties**
- **Ensure safety for all**
- **Protect against contamination**
- **Be calm and confident**
- **Ensure that the appropriate emergency services have been called for**

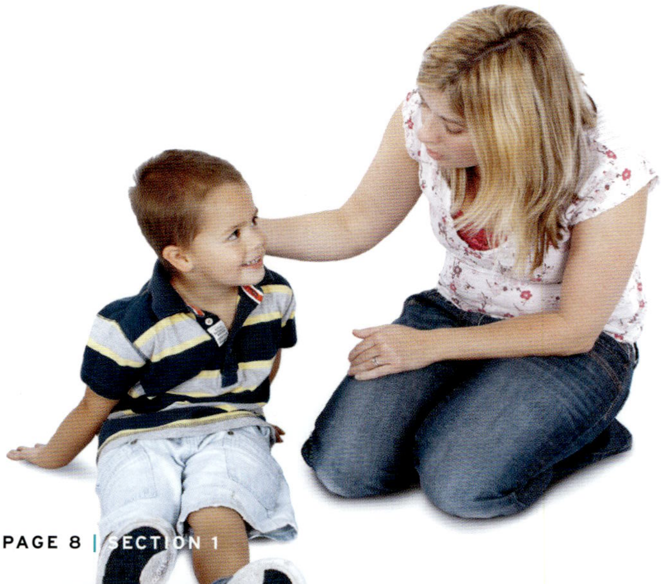

CASUALTY COMMUNICATION

Irrespective of the severity of the incident, your casualty could be in a state of shock and confusion. Therefore, your communication skills are critical in gaining their trust.

The groups that are most likely to be affected are children, the elderly, hearing impaired, visually impaired and non-English speaking casualties.

- **Be honest about their condition, without exaggerating it**
- **Be careful of what you say which could distress them further**
- **Maintain eye contact when talking to them, and be aware of your body language. Their body language could tell you a lot about their condition**
- **Take your time when talking to them, particularly for the vulnerable groups such as the elderly and children**
- **Allow your casualty to explain how they are feeling. It could help you make a diagnosis enabling you to offer the right treatment**
- **In respect of their injury, avoid medical terms that they may not understand**
- **Explain to the parents or guardians what is being done**
- **Provide a child with a comforter such as a toy or their blanket**

L I O N E L

CONTACTING THE EMERGENCY SERVICES

As soon as you have identified the extent of the injury, then it may be necessary to contact the emergency services. They can be contacted by dialling 999 or 112.

They will require vital information about the condition of the casualty so that the call can be prioritised.

Activate the speaker function on the phone to aid communication with the ambulance service.

They will also require specific details about the location of the incident. It is imperative that you have the full details of where you are, particularly if the premises are large and have multi-floors or other buildings to consider. Your bystander could manage this for you by meeting the emergency services and guiding them to the incident.

Only dial 999 if it is necessary and consider other services such as the Police and Fire, dependent on the incident.

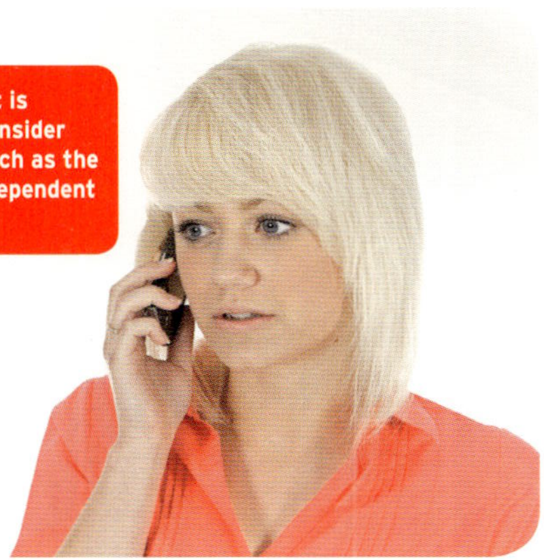

Remember **LIONEL** when making this call:

- **L** **Location**
- **I** **Incident**
- **O** **Other services**
- **N** **Number of casualties**
- **E** **Extent of injuries**
- **L** **Location - repeat**

PRIORITISE YOUR FIRST AID TREATMENT

- **Breathing** - deal with casualties who are not breathing normally first
- **Bleeding** - deal with any major bleeding and treat the casualty for shock
- **Burns/breaks** - treat burns and immobilise any bone injuries
- **Other conditions** - treat appropriately

There are many conditions that could be deemed as life-threatening which require medication, such as diabetes, asthma and anaphylaxis. Where possible, you can assist your casualty by offering them their own medication if they have it with them.

Remember your priorities. Ensure that their airway remains open and that they are breathing normally for themselves.

THE CLEARING UP PROCESS AND INFECTION CONTROL

You must minimise the risk of infection from the outset when dealing with any incident. This applies to you, the casualty, and any bystanders. Similarly, when the casualty has been treated it is vital that all soiled dressings etc, are disposed of correctly.

- **Wash your hands and wear disposable gloves**
- **Avoid coughing and sneezing over the wound, and avoid touching it**
- **Dispose of all soiled dressings, including gloves, in an appropriately marked (orange/yellow) plastic bag**
- **Dispose of sharp items, including syringes and needles, in a purpose made sharps bin and dispose of it appropriately. It may mean taking it to your local hospital for correct disposal**

Rescuers should take appropriate safety precautions where feasible, especially if the casualty is known to have a serious infection such as tuberculosis (TB) or severe acute respiratory distress syndrome (SARS).

During an outbreak of a highly infectious condition such as SARS, then protective precautions for the rescuer are essential.

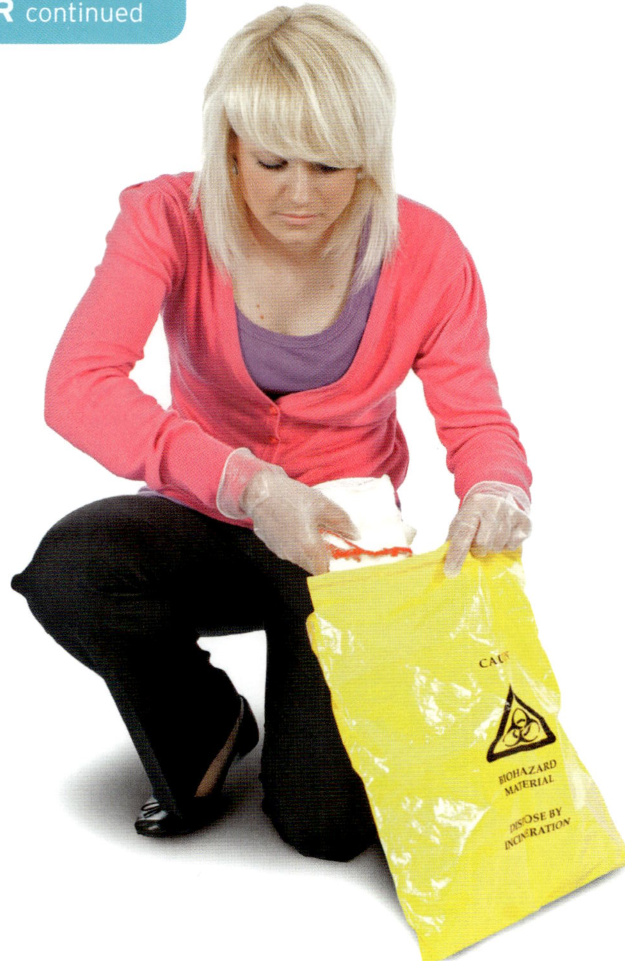

When confronted with any emergency situation, you need to take **SHAPE**!

S — Safety and protection

You must ensure the safety for all. Ensure you are adequately protected against the risk of infection and any other adverse element such as chemicals and gases

H — Hazards

Be aware of potential hazards such as traffic, chemicals, fire, gas, electricity etc

A — Assess the situation

Before rushing in to deal with an incident, you must assess the situation that you are confronted with

P — Prioritise

Ensure you prioritise the injuries, particularly if you have multiple casualties

E — Environment

Pay attention to the environment around you, and do not take risks. Jumping into water to save a drowning victim is not a good idea if you can't swim!

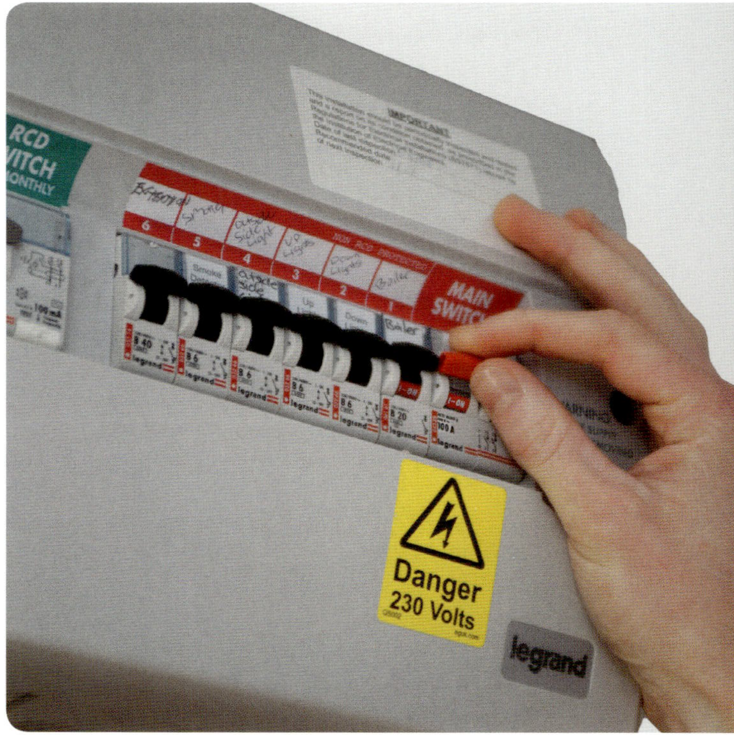

PRIMARY SURVEY

Irrespective of the incident you are confronted with, you must carry out an initial assessment of the situation including your casualty.

This is popularly known as the primary survey.

The contents of this survey can be remembered easily by using the mnemonic DR ABC.

D Dangers

The area must be safe before you offer your casualty any treatment. Safe for you primarily, not forgetting any bystanders and of course your casualty.

Failing to do this could result in you having more casualties to deal with, which could include yourself!

R Response

Approach the casualty, ideally from their feet.

This reduces the risk of the casualty hyper-extending their neck should they be responsive.

If they are responsive, ascertain the extent of their injury and deal with it appropriately.

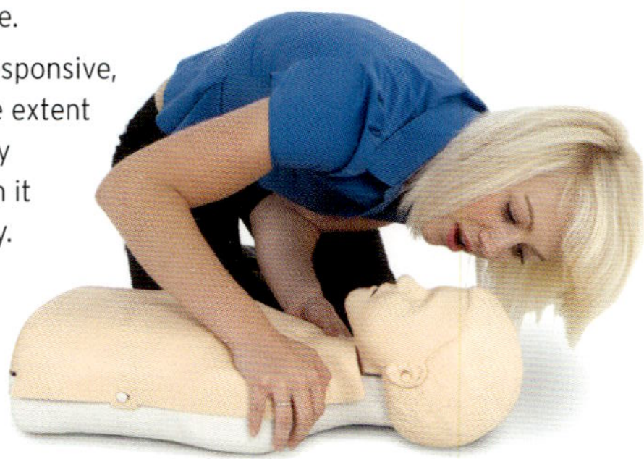

If they are not responsive, then:

- **Gently stimulate the child and ask loudly, 'Are you all right?'**
- **An infant can be stimulated by rubbing the soles of their feet with your finger**
- **Do not shake infants, or children with suspected cervical spine injuries**
- **Use their name when talking to them**

If they respond by answering or moving:

Leave them in the position in which you find them (provided they are not in further danger).

Check their condition, reassess them regularly and move on to your secondary assessment (page 15).

NB: If you need to make a telephone call, always endeavour to take the child or infant with you. Ideally they should not be left alone.

If there is no response at all, they must be deemed as being unresponsive or unresponsive.

If you are on your own, you should shout for help. Ideally, you should never leave your casualty on their own. A bystander can be a great benefit to you such as:

- **Calling for an ambulance**
- **Managing crowds and hazards**
- **Fetching the First Aid kit and defibrillator if you have one**
- **Consoling relatives and friends**
- **Helping you if they are trained to do so**
- **Cleaning up**
- **A support for you**

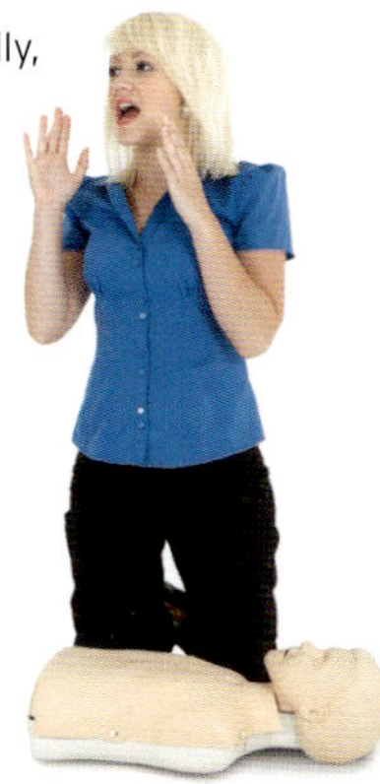

A

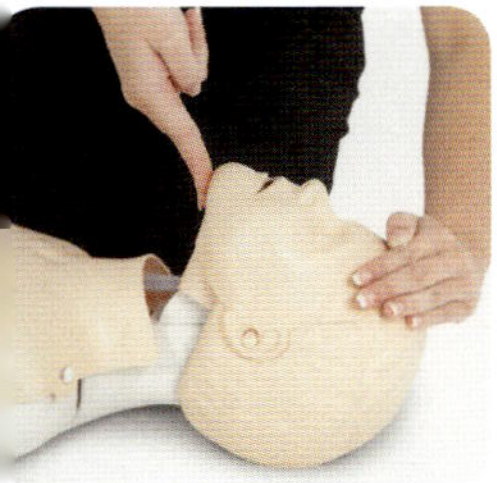

Airway

Turn the child/infant onto their back and open their airway using the head tilt and chin lift manoeuvre:

- **Place your hand on their forehead and gently tilt their head back. Be very careful not to over extend this movement with an infant**
- **With two fingertips under the point of their chin, lift the child's chin. Use one finger for an infant**

In either case, do not push on the soft tissues under the chin as this may block the airway.

B

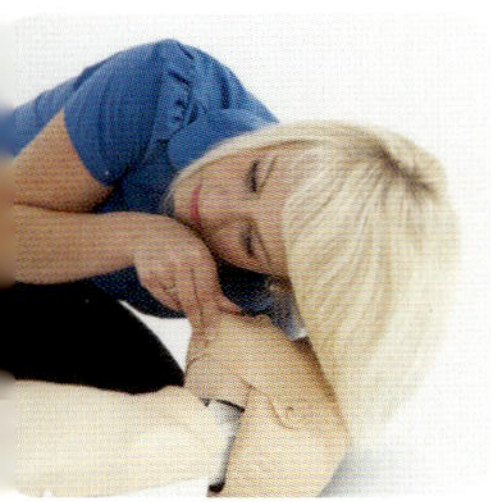

Breathing

Look, listen and feel for normal breathing for no more than 10 seconds.

Look for chest movement

Listen at their mouth for breath sounds

Feel for air on your cheek

In the first few minutes after cardiac arrest, a casualty may be barely breathing, or taking infrequent, noisy, gasps. This is often termed agonal breathing or gasping, and must not be confused with normal breathing. If you have any doubt whether breathing is normal, act as if it is not normal and prepare to commence CPR.

C

CPR for a non-breathing casualty

If their breathing is not normal or absent:

- **Send your bystander immediately to call for an ambulance and to return with a defibrillator, if one is available, whilst you commence CPR without delay** (See page 20)

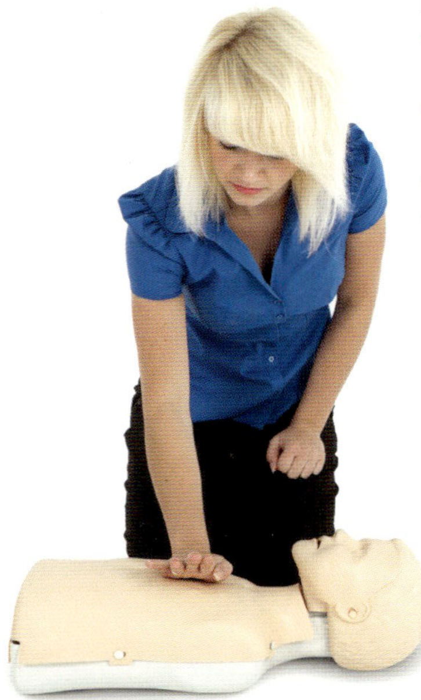

If you have no bystander, then:

- **Carefully remove any obvious airway obstruction**
- **Give 5 initial rescue breaths followed by 1 minute of CPR**
- **Call for an ambulance**
- **Continue with CPR**

If you are able to, activate the speaker function on your phone to aid communication between you and the emergency services.

The casualty who is **unresponsive** and not **breathing normally** is in cardiac arrest and requires CPR.

Immediately following cardiac arrest blood flow to the brain is reduced to virtually zero, which may cause seizure-like episodes that may be confused with epilepsy.

You should be suspicious of cardiac arrest with any casualty that presents seizure like symptoms and carefully assess whether they are breathing normally.

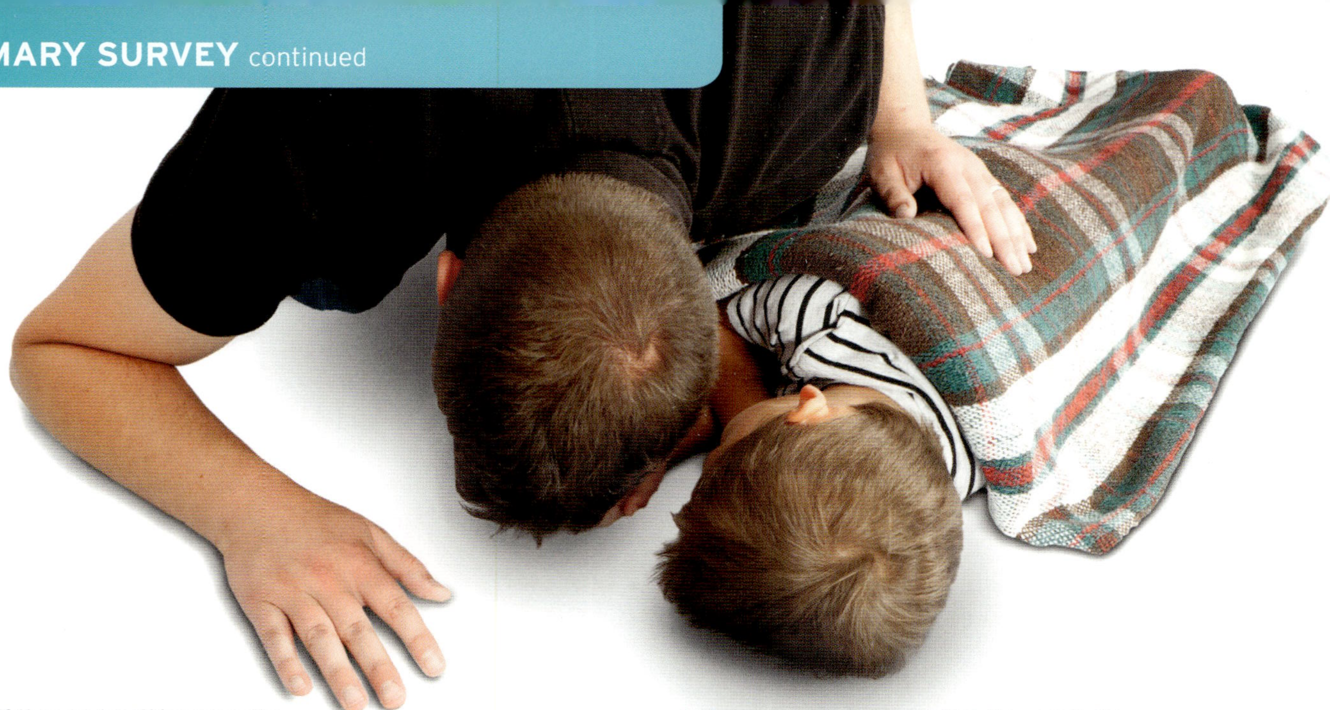

If they are breathing normally:

- **Treat any injuries accordingly and put them in the recovery position (see page 16)**
- **Ask your bystander to summon an ambulance. If you are on your own, then make this call yourself taking the casualty with you if it's possible. Maintain an open airway by holding them in the recovery position. If it's not possible, place them in the recovery position in order to maintain an open airway before leaving them**
- **Upon your return ensure that they are in the recovery position and monitor their breathing until the emergency services take over from you.** Should they stop breathing normally, then start CPR (see page 20)

If you are unsure about the extent of the injury, then try to make a diagnosis based upon the signs that you can see, the symptoms that the casualty is feeling and the history, before placing them in the recovery position (see page 16).

SECONDARY ASSESSMENT

As soon as you have completed your primary survey, and you have established that your casualty is breathing normally, you must then move on to the secondary assessment in order to determine the extent of their injury or illness, irrespective of whether they are responsive or not.

In order to make a diagnosis of their condition, there are three key factors to consider. By making this diagnosis correctly, it should determine the treatment you offer them. In all cases, your priority is to maintain an open airway and to ensure that they are breathing normally.

History

- **Ask your casualty or bystanders what happened**
- **Examine the environment for obvious signs relating to the incident**
- **Ask your casualty about their condition. Do they have their own medication? Has it happened before? Where does it hurt? How painful is it?**
- **Ask the casualty their name. Is there any family present that could answer the questions about their condition?**

Signs

- **What can you see in respect of the injury or condition?**
- **Use all your other senses. What can you smell, hear and feel?**

Symptoms

This is how the casualty will be feeling, ask them how they are feeling.

- **Communication is very important to ascertain the extent of their injury/illness**
- **Continue to question their well-being throughout your assessment as they may have deteriorated which may influence your decision on the appropriate treatment**

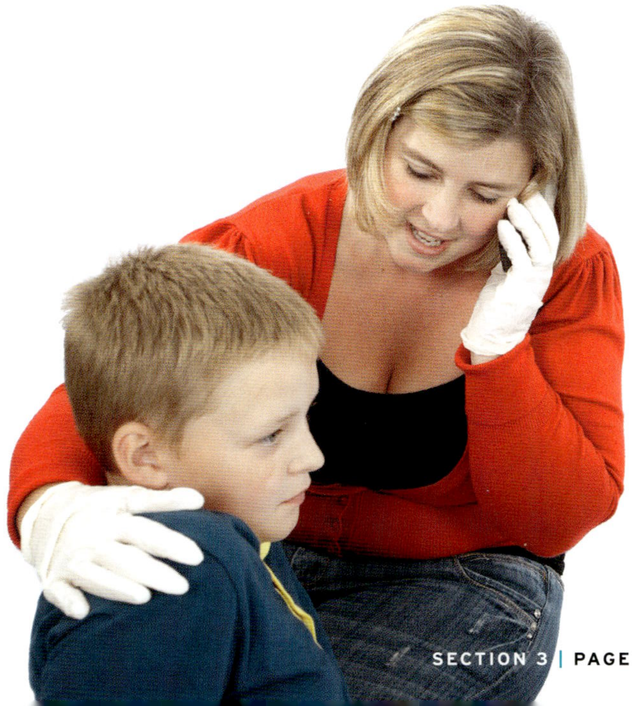

THE RECOVERY POSITION FOR A CHILD

If your casualty is unresponsive, but breathing normally, then your priority is to ensure that their airway is not compromised in any way and that it remains open.

Rather than leaving them on their back, or in a slumped position, then an effective way of achieving this is to place them in the recovery position.

Whilst the casualty remains in this position, it will allow vomit to drain from the mouth and prevent them from rolling onto their back should you have to leave them.

1. **Remove the casualty's glasses, if present**
2. **Kneel beside the casualty and make sure that both their legs are straight**
3. **Place the arm nearest to you out at a right angle to their body, elbow bent with the hand palm-up. Do not force the arm, let it fall naturally, but close to this position**

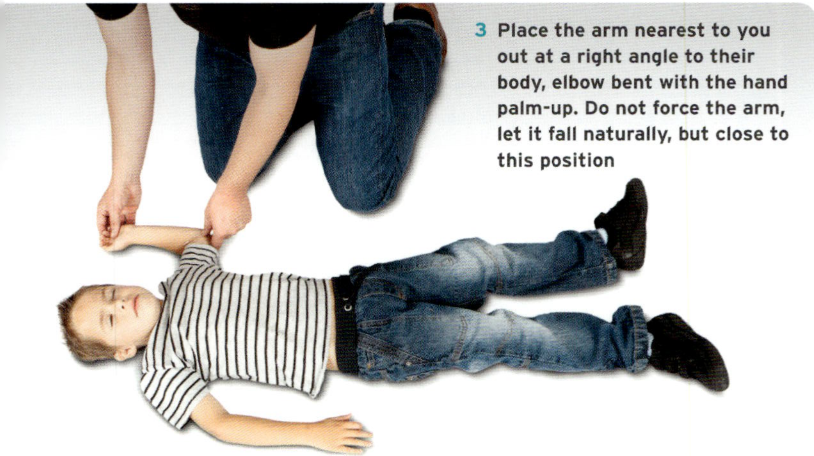

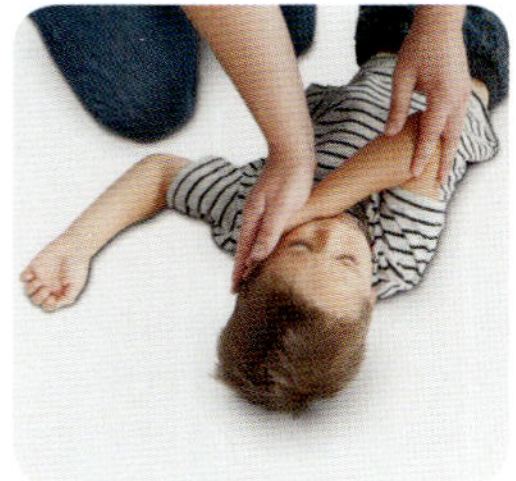

4. **Bring the far arm across the chest, and hold the back of the hand against their cheek nearest to you**

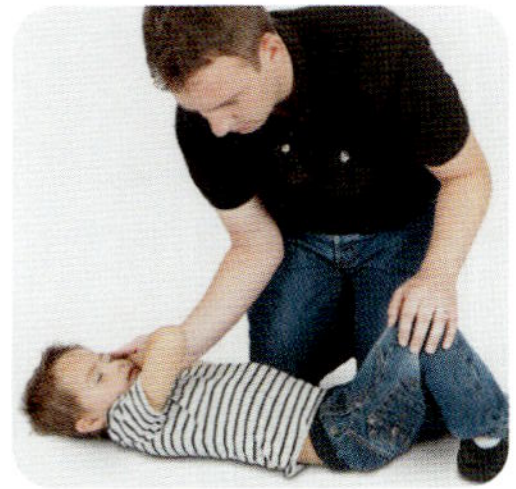

5. **Grab hold of the far leg with your other hand, and raise the knee so that their foot is kept to the floor. This will be your lever for rolling them over**

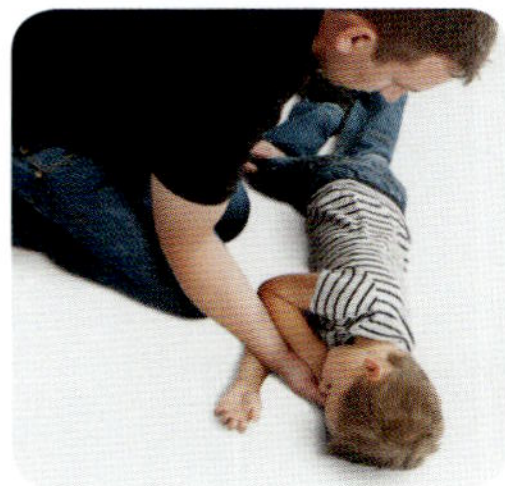

6. **Keeping their hand pressed against their cheek, pull on the far leg to roll them towards you onto their side with their head supported all the way**

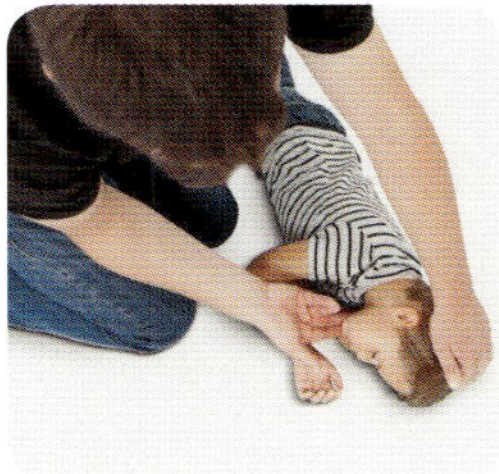

7 **Tilt the head back to make sure that the airway remains open**

8 **Adjust the upper leg so that both the hip and knee are bent at right angles**

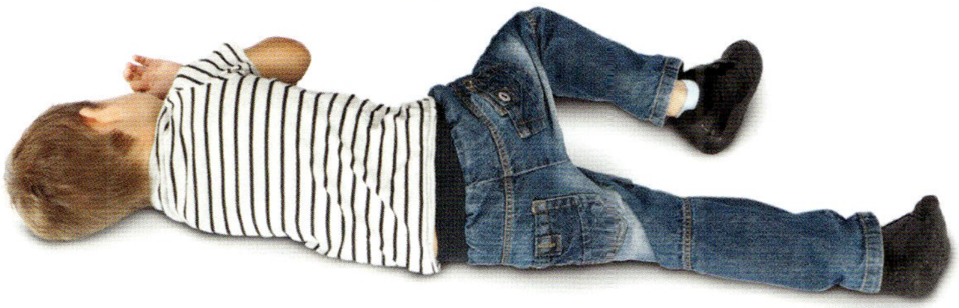

9 **If you have a bystander available to you, then this is the time to send them to call for an ambulance ensuring they have all the appropriate information, and in particular, the condition of the casualty**

10 **If you have no bystander, you must call for an ambulance yourself**

If they have to be kept in the recovery position for **more than 30 minutes** turn them to the opposite side to relieve the pressure on the lower arm.

You must continue to monitor their breathing whilst waiting for the emergency services to take over. If they stop breathing normally, then you must call the emergency services with an update and commence CPR immediately.

It will also be worth monitoring and noting other changes such as colouration of the skin, their temperature and responsiveness levels.

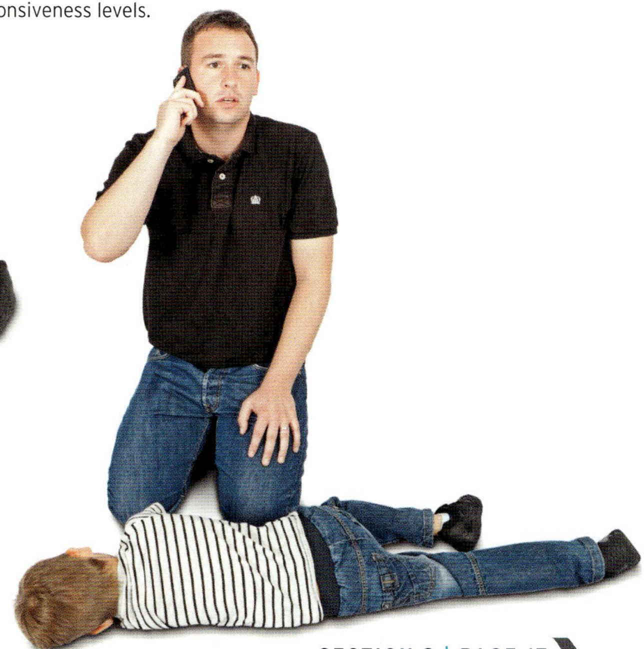

THE RECOVERY POSITION FOR AN INFANT

If the infant is unresponsive, but breathing normally, then your priority is to ensure that their airway is not compromised in any way and that it remains open.

Rather than leaving them on their back, an effective way of achieving this is to place them in the recovery position.

Hold the infant in your arms with their head facing downwards and towards you so that you can monitor their airway, their breathing and their general condition.

If their condition deteriorates in any way, then it is vital to update the emergency services.

It is important to keep them with you at all times, particularly when contacting the emergency services.

Whilst the casualty remains in this position, it will allow vomit to drain from their mouth and maintain an open airway.

If their breathing stops or it is not normal, then:

- **Send your bystander immediately to call for an ambulance whilst you commence CPR without delay**

If you have no bystander, then:

- **Carefully remove any obvious airway obstruction**
- **Give 5 initial rescue breaths followed by 1 minute of CPR**
- **Call for an ambulance**
- **Continue with CPR**

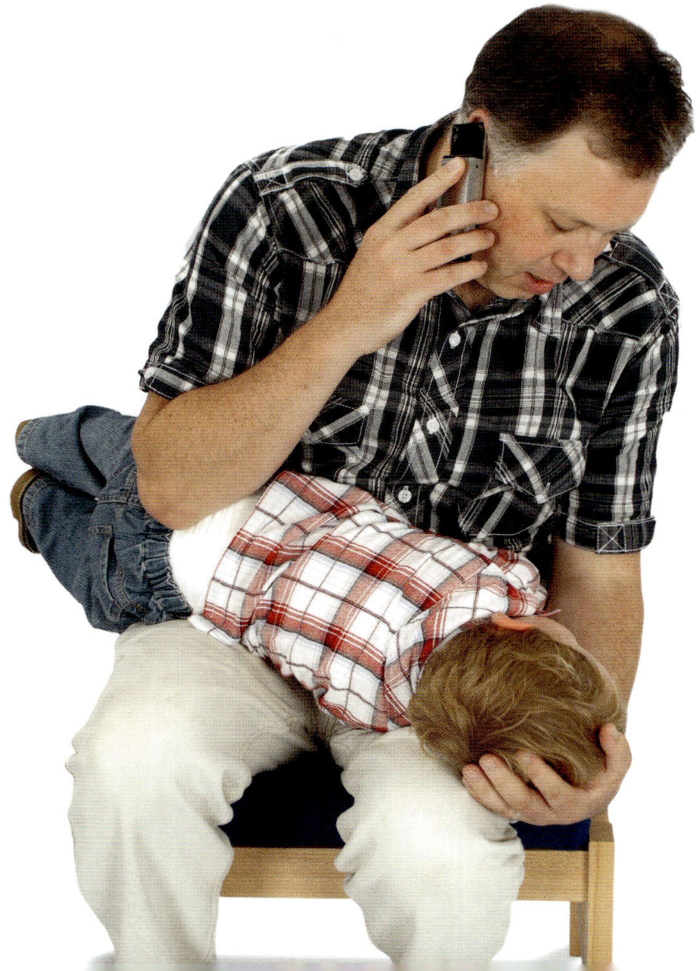

THE RESPIRATORY SYSTEM

Our ability to breathe is thanks to our respiratory system which is made up primarily of our airways and our lungs.

We are able to breathe in and out spontaneously providing we have air to breathe and the airways are open.

COMPOSITION OF AIR

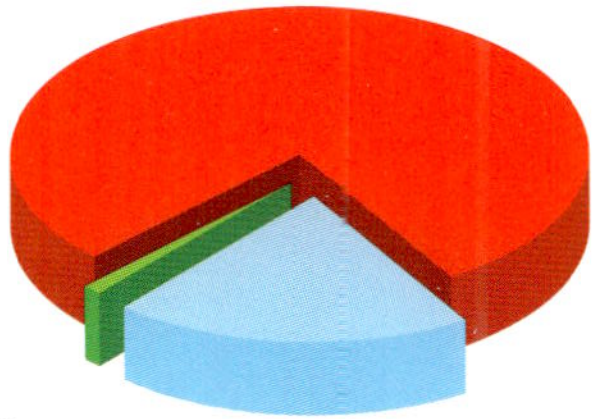

When we breathe in the diaphragm contracts and flattens, the ribs are elevated, and as negative pressure is produced in the chest cavity, there is increased pressure in the abdomen.
This draws air into the lungs to equalise the pressure.

We exhale when the diaphragm relaxes and the chest wall and lung tissue returns to their original size.

Respiration is achieved through the mouth, nose, trachea, lungs, and diaphragm. Oxygen enters the respiratory system through the mouth and the nose. The oxygen then passes through the larynx (where speech sounds are produced) and the trachea which is a tube that enters the chest cavity. In the chest cavity, the trachea splits into two smaller tubes called the bronchi. Each bronchus then divides again forming the bronchioles. These bronchial tubes lead directly into the lungs where they divide into many smaller tubes which connect to tiny sacs called alveoli. The average adult's lungs contain about 600 million of these spongy, air-filled sacs that are surrounded by capillaries. The inhaled oxygen passes into the alveoli and then enters the capillaries (diffusion) into the arterial blood which is taken back to the heart for circulating around the body.

Meanwhile, the waste-rich blood from the veins releases its carbon dioxide into the alveoli. The carbon dioxide follows the same path out of the lungs when you breathe out.

Approximately 25% of the available oxygen in each breath is used, as our body can only cope with so much each time we breathe in.

Carbon dioxide and other non-essential gases are breathed out, and the whole process is repeated approximately:

30-40 times for an infant under the age of 1
25-35 times for a child 1-2 years of age
25-30 times for a child 2-5 years of age
20-25 times for a child 5-12 years of age
10-20 times for someone > 12 years of age

The Respiratory System

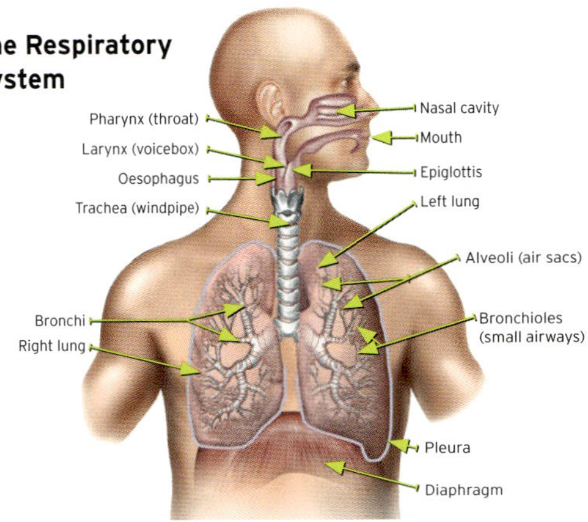

RESUSCITATION AND AED

Cardiopulmonary resuscitation (CPR) is an emergency procedure which is attempted in an effort to return life to a child or infant who is not breathing normally for themselves.

This procedure combines chest compressions with rescue breaths. The chest compression replaces the heart's ability to pump oxygenated blood around the body, particularly the vital organs such as the brain.

Rescue breathing provides the casualty, who is unable to breathe normally for themselves, valuable oxygen that is transported around the body in the bloodstream by the chest compressions.

Without oxygen, brain damage can occur within three minutes. Therefore, your immediate action is paramount.

Referring back to Primary Survey, ie: DR ABC, you will have established that your casualty is not breathing normally.

Your immediate action now is to send your bystander to call the emergency services for an ambulance, ensuring they have the correct information, with particular reference that your casualty is not breathing normally.

- **Carefully remove any airway obstruction**
- **Give 5 initial rescue breaths**
- **Give 30 chest compressions followed by a further 2 rescue breaths**
- **Repeat the sequence 30:2**

If you don't have a bystander, then you must administer 5 initial breaths, followed by 1 minute of CPR (approximately 2 cycles of 30 chest compressions followed by 2 breaths) before contacting the emergency services yourself.

Continue with CPR (30:2) until the emergency services take over from you, your casualty recovers* or you become too exhausted to continue.

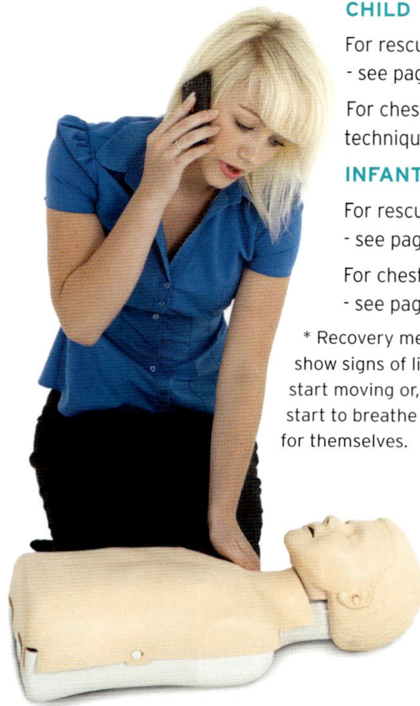

CHILD

For rescue breath technique - see page 21

For chest compression technique - see page 23

INFANT

For rescue breath technique - see page 22

For chest compression technique - see page 24

* Recovery means that they start to show signs of life i.e. they wake up or, start moving or, open their eyes **and** they start to breathe normally for themselves.

Defibrillation

If you have an Automated External Defibrillator (AED) available to you, you should immediately unpack it, attach the pads, switch it on and follow the voice prompts.

(Please see pages 25-29 for further information).

TECHNIQUE FOR GIVING RESCUE BREATHS FOR A CHILD OVER 1 YEAR:

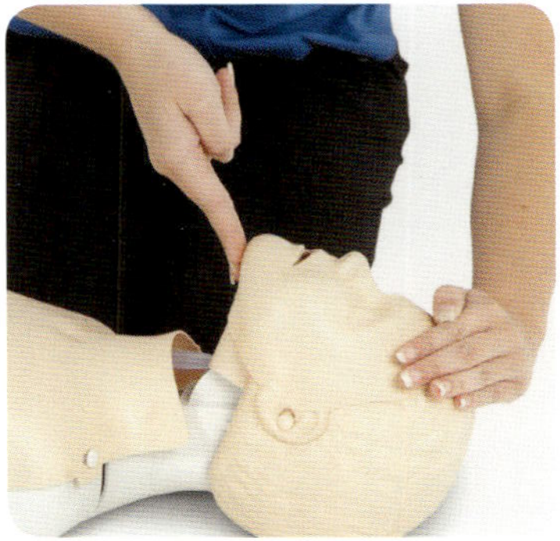

- Ensure head tilt and chin lift
- Pinch the soft part of their nose closed with the index finger and thumb of your hand on their forehead

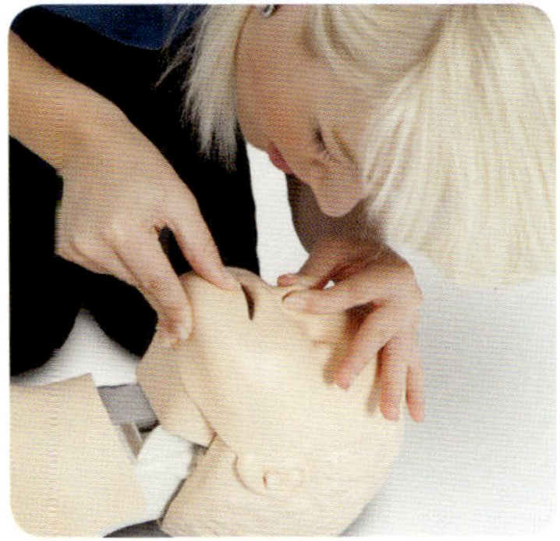

- Open their mouth a little, but maintain the chin lift
- Take a breath and place your lips around their mouth, making sure that you have a good seal

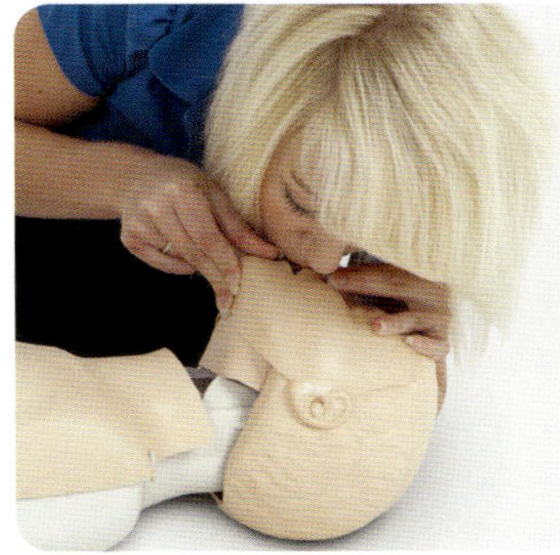

- Blow steadily into their mouth over 1 second, sufficient to make the chest rise visibly. This is the same time period as in adult practice
- Maintaining head tilt and chin lift, take your mouth away and watch for their chest to fall as air comes out
- Take another breath and repeat this sequence four more times. Identify the effectiveness by seeing that their chest has risen and fallen in a similar fashion to the movement produced by a normal breath

TECHNIQUE FOR GIVING RESCUE BREATHS FOR AN INFANT:

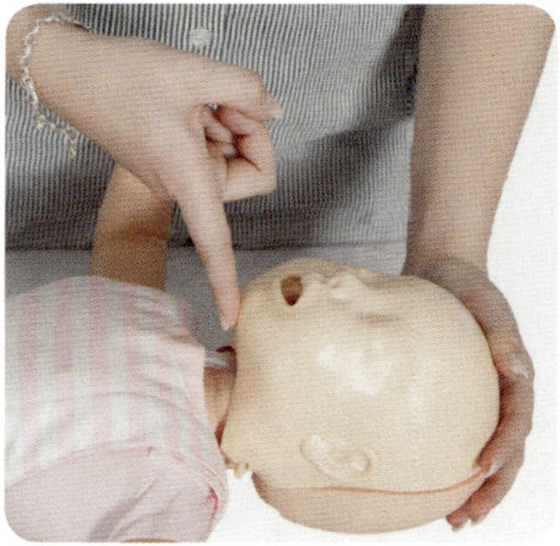

- Ensure a neutral position of the head (as an infant's head is usually flexed when on their back and face up (supine), this may require some extension) and apply chin lift
- Take a breath and cover the mouth and nose of the infant with your mouth, making sure you have a good seal. If both the nose and mouth cannot be covered in the older infant, then attempt to seal only the infant's nose or mouth with your mouth (if the nose is used, close the lips to prevent air escape and vice versa)

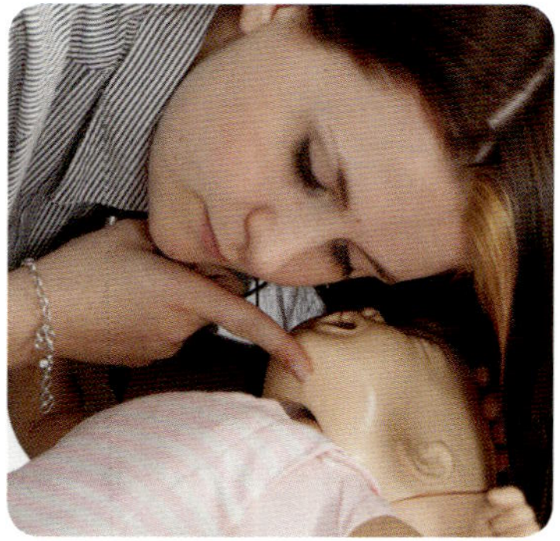

- Blow steadily into their mouth over 1 second, sufficient to make the chest rise visibly. This is the same time period as in adult practice
- Maintain head position and chin lift, take your mouth away, and watch for their chest to fall as air comes out
- Identify the effectiveness by seeing that their chest has risen and fallen in a similar fashion to the movement produced by a normal breath

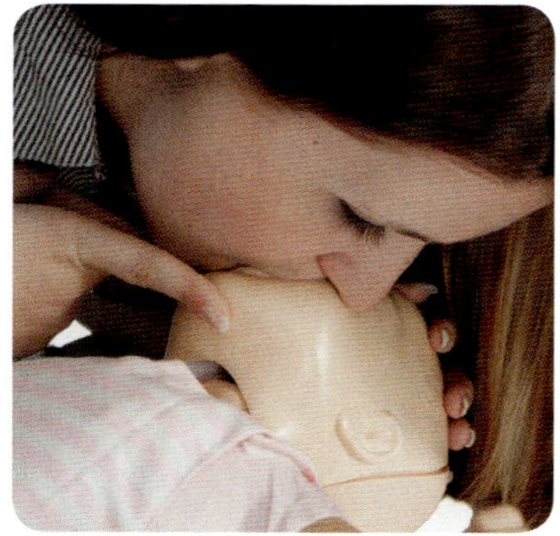

For both infants and children, if you have difficulty achieving an effective breath, the airway may be obstructed:

- Open their mouth and remove any visible obstruction. Do not perform a blind finger sweep
- Ensure that there is adequate head tilt and chin lift but also that the neck is not over extended
- Make up to 5 attempts to achieve effective breaths. If this is still unsuccessful, move on to chest compressions

TECHNIQUE FOR GIVING CHEST COMPRESSIONS FOR CHILDREN AGED OVER 1 YEAR:

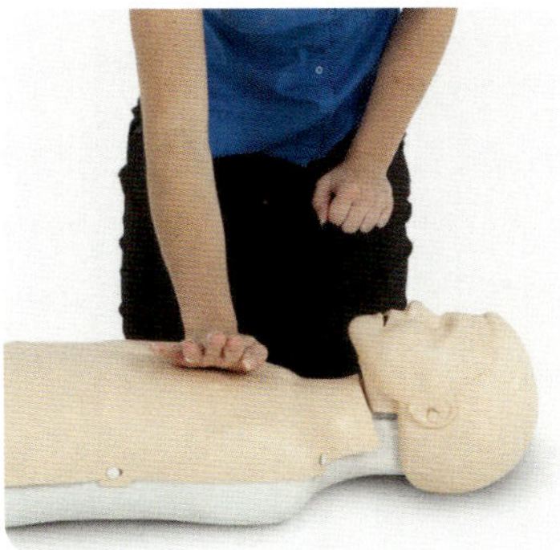

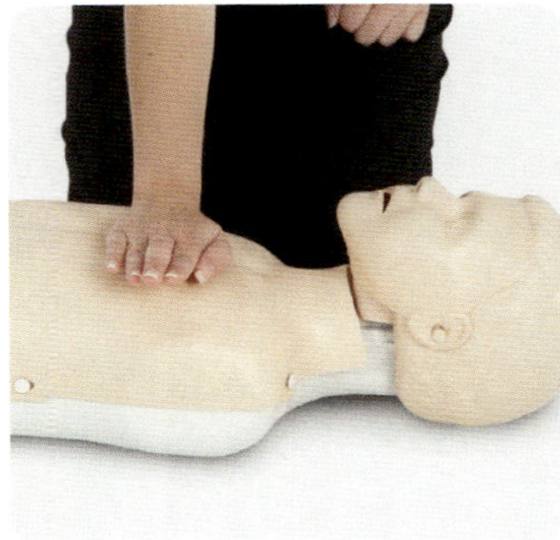

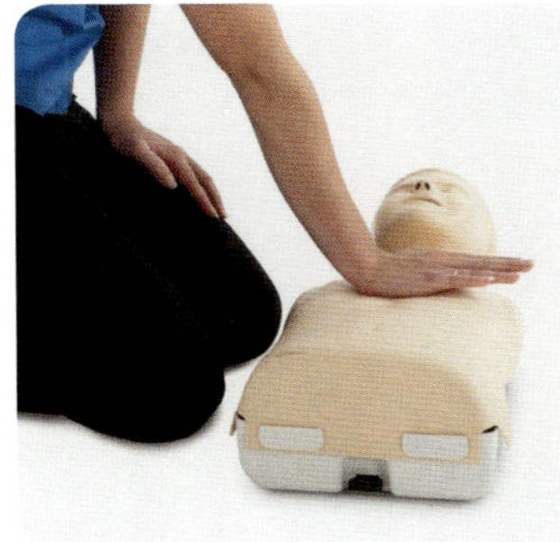

- **Place the heel of one hand on the lower half of the breastbone (sternum)**
- **Lift the fingers to ensure that pressure is not applied over their ribs**
- **Position yourself vertically above their chest and, with your arm straight, compress the sternum to depress it by at least one-third of the depth of the chest, which is approximately 5cms, and at a speed of 100-120 compressions per minute. For larger children, or for small rescuers, this may be achieved more easily by using both hands with the fingers interlocked**

After giving 30 chest compressions, give 2 rescue breaths.

Repeat the sequence of 30:2.

Continue with CPR (30:2) until the emergency services take over from you, your casualty recovers* or you become too exhausted to continue.

* Recovery means that they start to show signs of life i.e. they wake up, or start moving, or open their eyes **and** they start to breathe normally for themselves.

RESUSCITATION AND AED continued

TECHNIQUE FOR GIVING CHEST COMPRESSIONS FOR INFANTS:

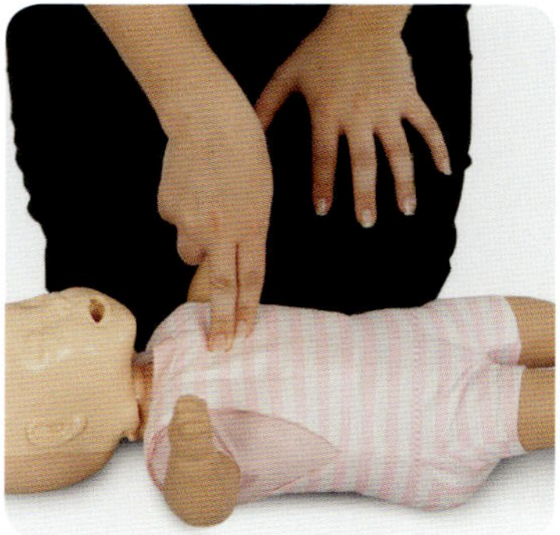

- **Place the tips of 2 fingers in the centre of the breastbone (sternum)**
- **Compress the sternum to depress it by at least one-third of the depth of the chest which is approximately 4cms**
- **Release the pressure completely, then repeat at a rate of 100-120 compressions per Minute**

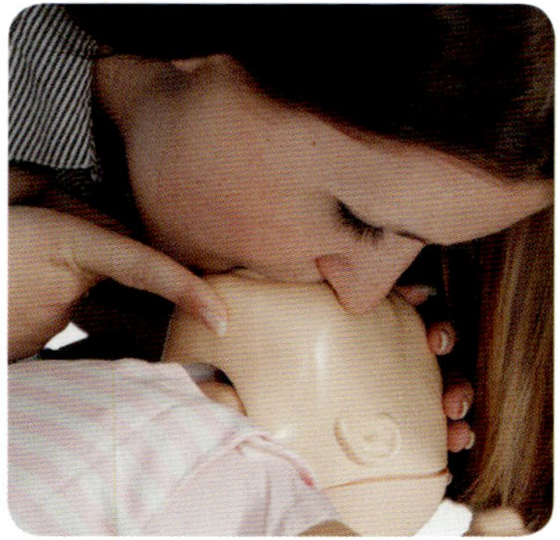

- **After giving 30 chest compressions, give 2 rescue breaths**
- **Repeat the sequence of 30:2**
- **Continue with CPR (30:2) until the emergency services take over from you, your casualty recovers* or you become too exhausted to continue**

* Recovery means that they start to show signs of life i.e. they wake up, or start moving, or open their eyes **and** they start to breathe normally for themselves.

DEFIBRILLATION WITH AN AED

In the rare event a child needs defibrillating, follow these guidelines as detailed on Pages 25 - 28 but pay particular attention to Page 29 where specific information can be found on paediatric pads.

The resuscitation procedure for a child will be the same as detailed earlier.

If your casualty is in a wet environment, then move them to a dry area and ensure that they are not in contact with anything metal.

When the AED arrives, you must immediately unpack it and prepare to fix the pads to the casualty. If you have trained help, then allow them to continue with CPR until you are ready. If not, then stop CPR and unpack it yourself.

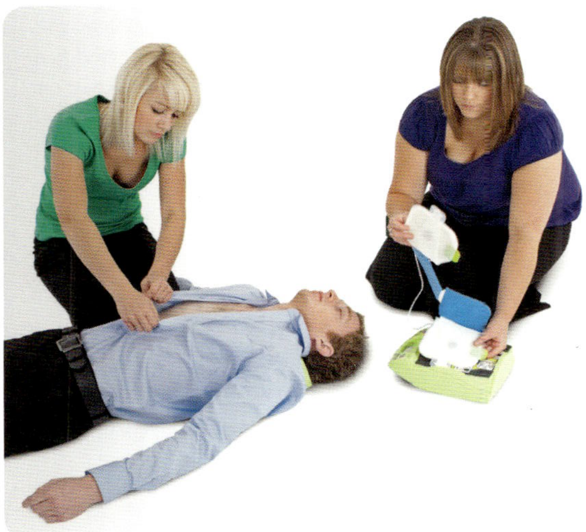

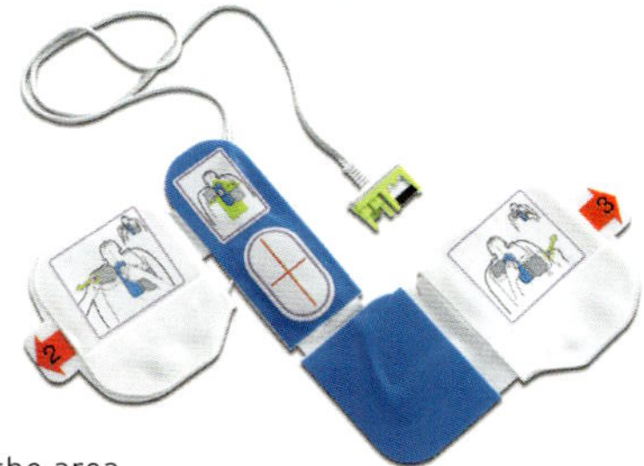

If your casualty is wearing a wired bra, then this must be removed or cut through to expose the chest, particularly the area where the pads are to be fixed. Similarly, if your casualty is wearing jewellery that may come into contact with the pads, then it must be removed.

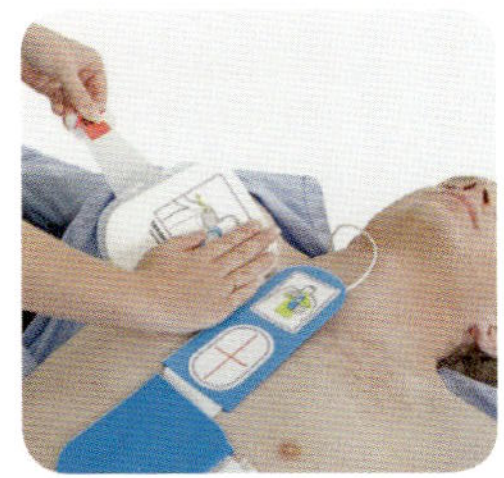

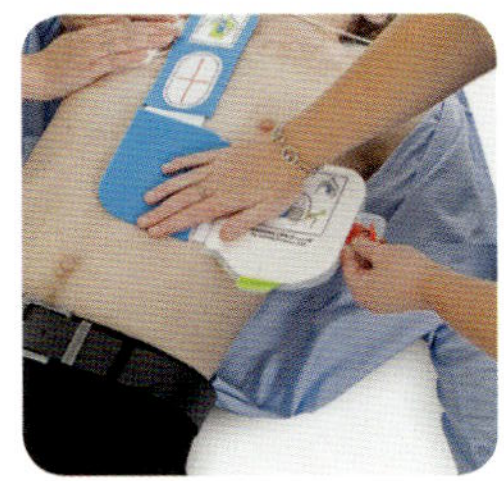

The majority of pads will be clearly marked on where they should be fixed. Depending on the make and model of the AED, the pads will generally come as two separate pads. Some will come as a single pad. Ensure that the film that is protecting the sticky pads is removed.

If your casualty has a pacemaker fitted, then ensure that the pads are placed at least 10cms away from it.

Do not place the pads directly on top of it. A pacemaker should be clearly identifiable, from a scar or what appears to be a small plate under the skin.

It may be necessary to prepare the casualty's chest in order for the pads to adhere. Do not waste valuable time shaving inappropriately.

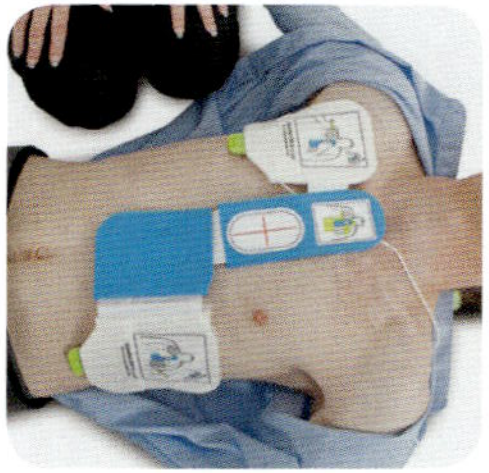

Most AED pads are labelled left and right, or carry a picture of the placement. It does not matter if these pads are reversed. What is important is that should they be placed the wrong way round, they must be left in place because the adhesive may well be removed or compromised if you swap them around.

In respect of switching the AED on, they will vary from one AED to another. Some will switch themselves on as soon as the lid is removed or opened. Others will have a button to press to switch it on.

It is important that you familiarise yourself with the AED you have.

All AED's will have a voice prompt and it is important that you follow these prompts.

Some AED's will also have a screen giving you the commands. This can be a very useful aid for those who are hard of hearing.

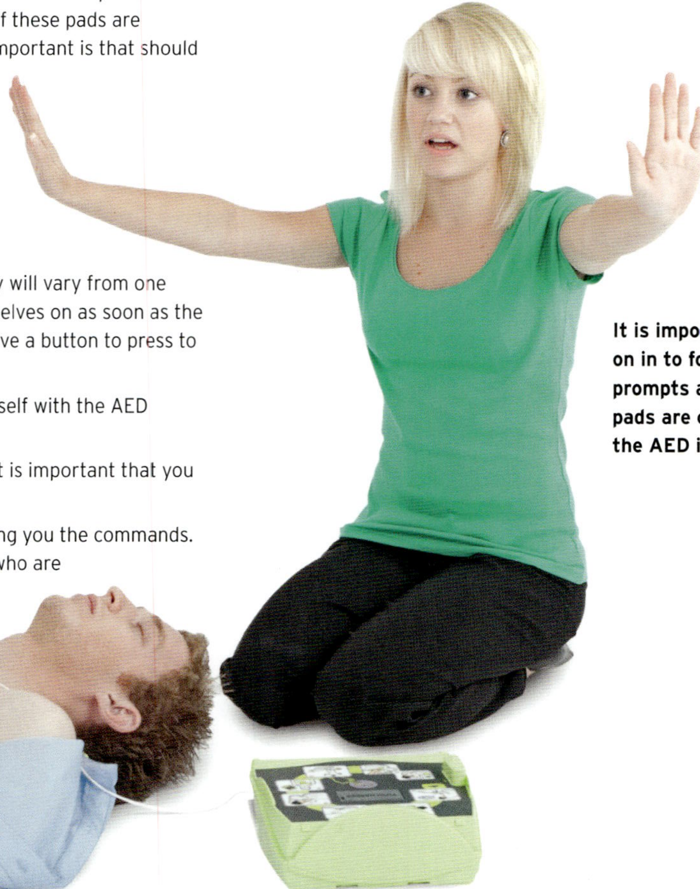

It is important from here on in to follow these prompts as soon as the pads are connected and the AED is switched on.

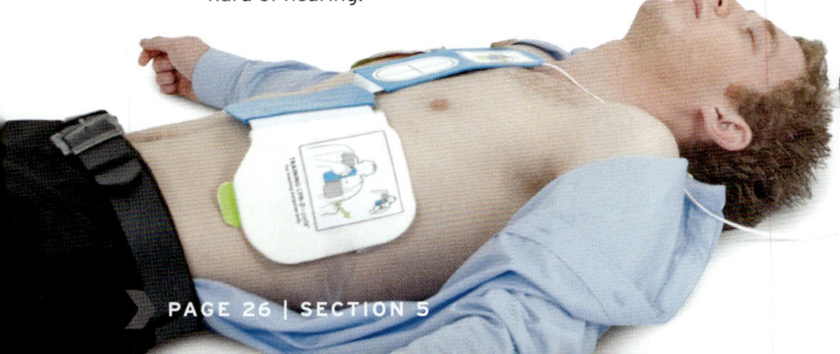

The AED will need to analyse the heart's rhythm. You will be prompted to ensure that no-one is touching the casualty, including yourself. Anyone touching the casualty could have an adverse effect on detecting the correct rhythm of your casualty's heart.

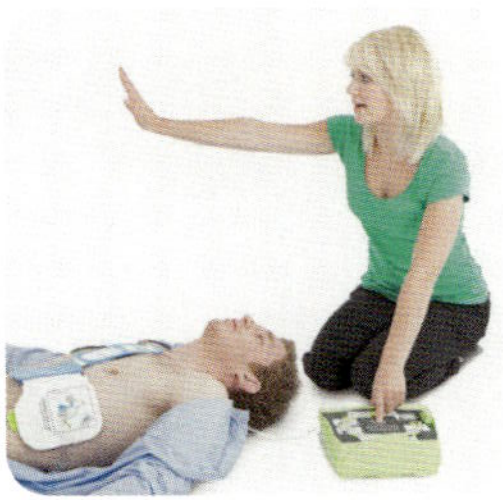

Dependent on the model you have, analysis will automatically happen, or you may have to push the 'Analyse' button.

You have to take control of the situation and move people away from the casualty.

Your next prompt could be to shock the casualty. Your AED may do this automatically, or you may have to press the 'Shock' button.

Again, manage the situation and ensure that no-one is touching the casualty.

Keep following the prompts from the AED.

If you are prompted to commence CPR, then quality CPR is important.

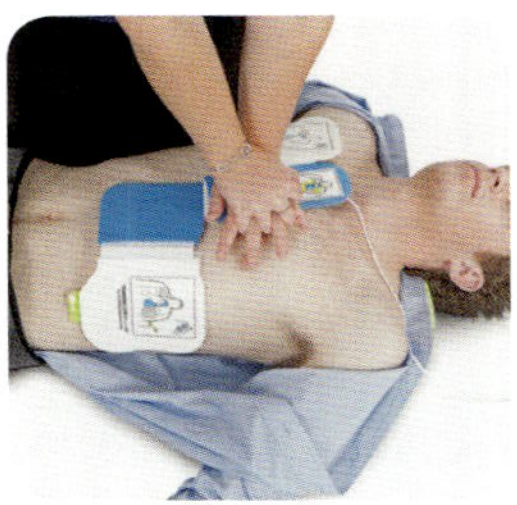

Ensure that you compress the chest at the right depth (dependent on age), and at the right speed of 100-120 chest compressions per minute.

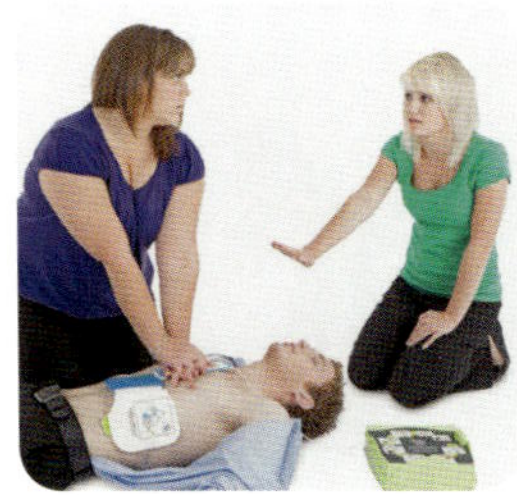

In essence you must continue with CPR until the AED tells you to stop to either analyse the casualty's heart rhythm, or it decides that a shock should be given.

Under the current 2015 Resuscitation guidelines, you will be administering CPR for two minutes before the AED will prompt you to stop in order for it to analyse the heart's rhythm.

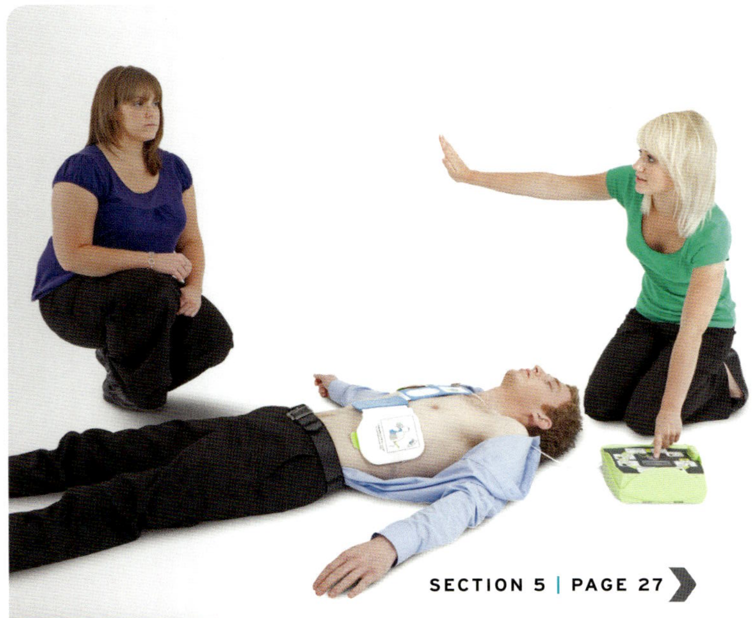

RESUSCITATION AND AED continued

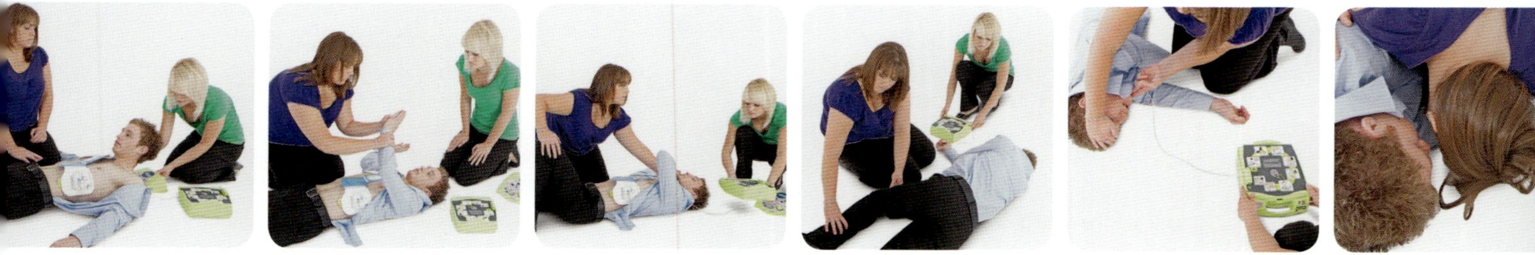

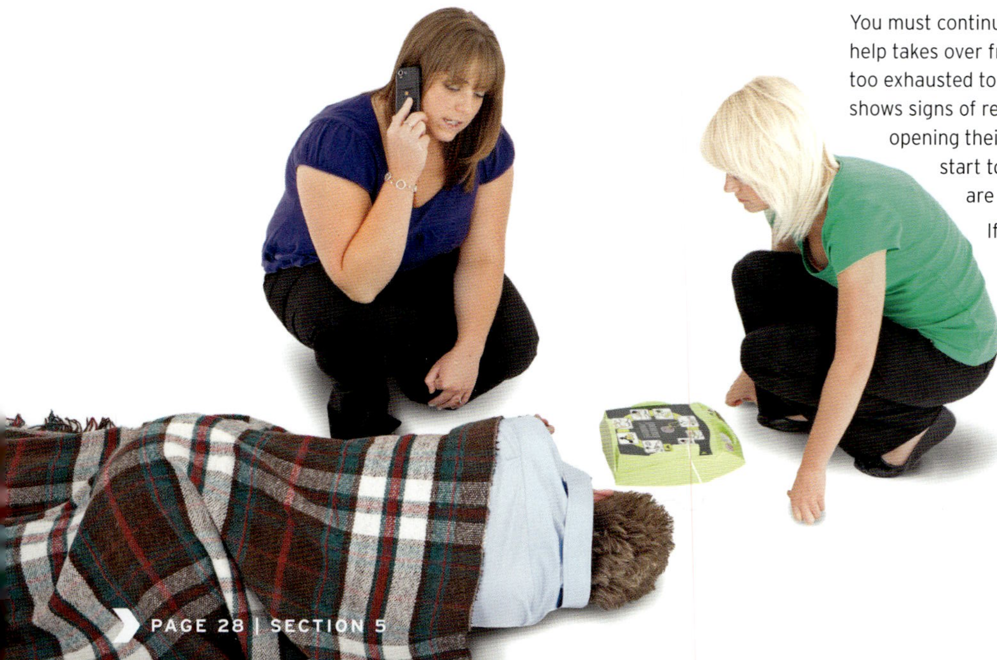

You must continue to follow the prompts until professional medical help takes over from you, your casualty recovers, or you become too exhausted to continue. Recovery will mean that your casualty shows signs of regaining responsiveness, such as coughing, opening their eyes, speaking or moving purposefully AND they start to breathe normally for themselves. To ensure they are breathing normally, conduct a breathing check.

If you are confident that they are breathing normally, place them in the recovery position with the pads attached and connected to the AED.

You must continue to monitor their breathing until professional medical help arrives and takes over from you.

PAEDIATRIC DEFIBRILLATION

The protocol for paediatric defibrillation is the same as that for an adult.

Most manufacturers are able to offer you specially modified pads for children, that means you can use the same AED for adults and children. However, what it is important to know are the differences between adults, children and infants in respect of your Basic Life Support procedures. This section deals with those differences.

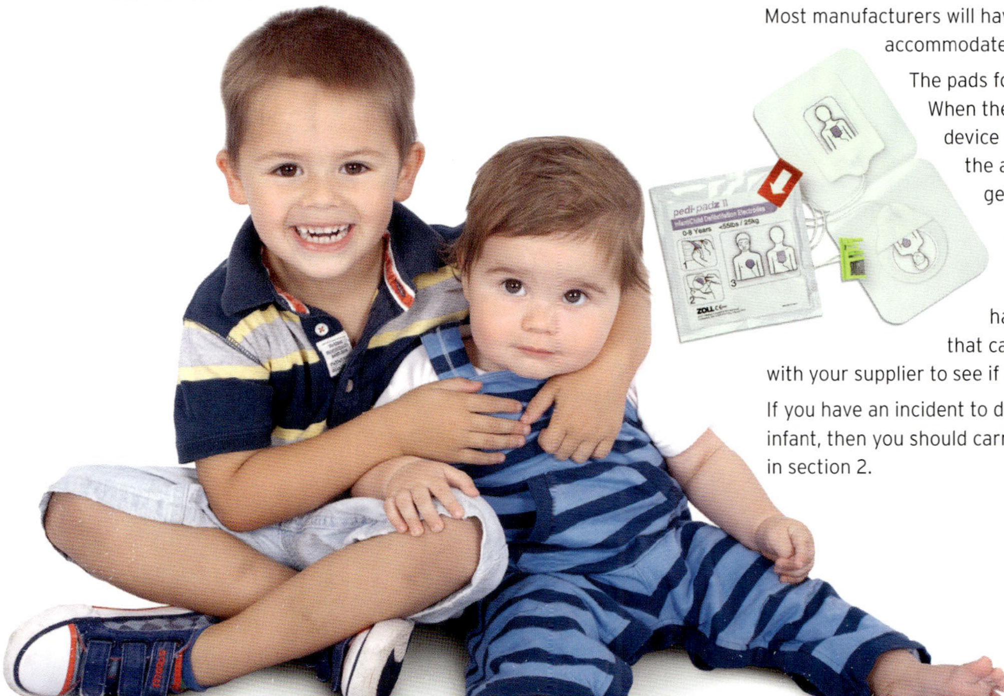

The term paediatric refers to children and infants (babies). A child is deemed as being aged from 1 to the onset of puberty and an infant being aged under 1 year old.

Many manufacturers refer to children as being from the age of 1 to 8. If you are in doubt about whether a child has reached puberty, then use the age of 8 as your guide. Any child that is older than 8 years of age should be treated as an adult, and the adult protocols for CPR and defibrillation should be adopted.

Most manufacturers will have specially adapted pads to accommodate a child.

The pads for children are generally smaller. When they are connected to the AED, the device will recognise them and administer the appropriate electric shock, which is generally a reduced charge.

Defibrillation is not recommended for infants unless the manufacturer of the AED you have has specially adapted pads that can be connected. You must check with your supplier to see if pads are available.

If you have an incident to deal with that involves a child or infant, then you should carry out a primary survey as defined in section 2.

THE CHAIN OF SURVIVAL

It is critical that you follow this chain when you are dealing with a casualty who is not breathing normally.

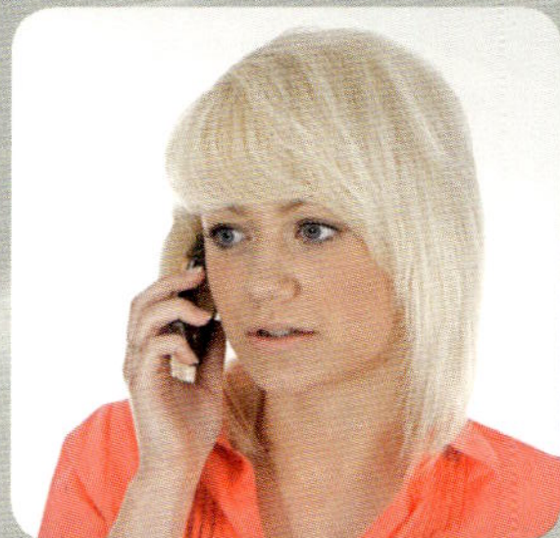

Early recognition and call for help

Recognise those at risk of cardiac arrest, and call for help in the hope that early treatment can prevent arrest.

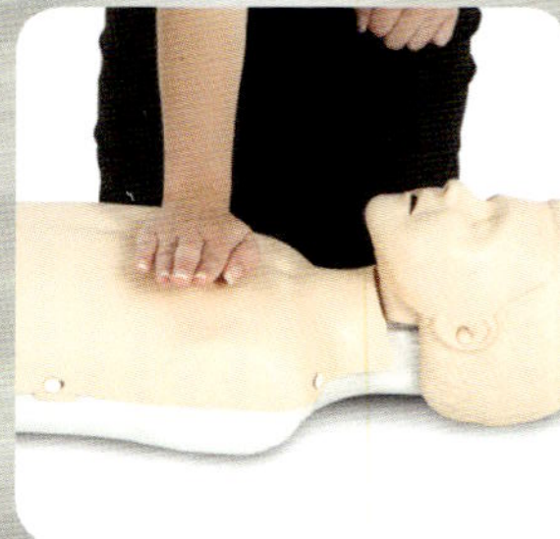

Early CPR

Start CPR to buy time until medical help arrives.

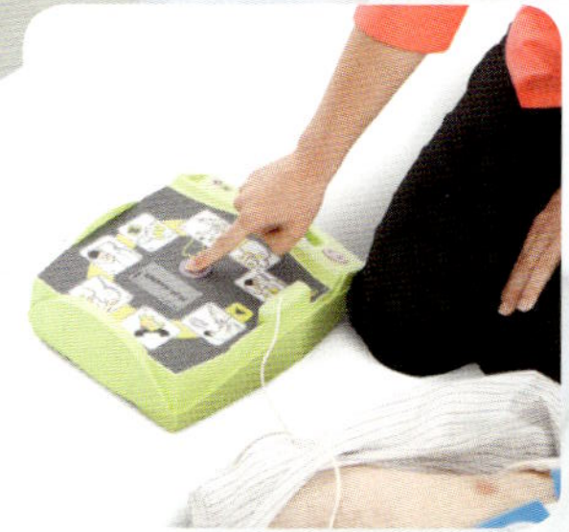

Early defibrillation

Defibrillators give an electric shock to re-organise the rhythm of the heart.

Defibrillation within 3-5 minutes of cardiac arrest can produce survival rates as high as 50-70%.

Each minute of delay to defibrillation reduces the probability of survival to hospital discharge by 10%.

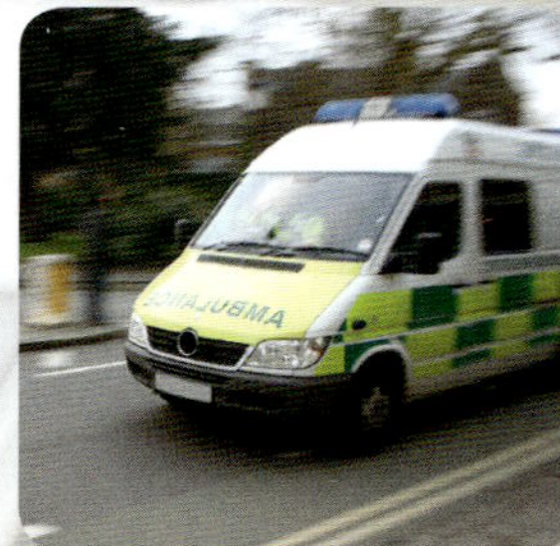

Post resuscitation care

Provide professional help in order to restore the quality of life.

SEIZURES

WHAT IS EPILEPSY?

Epilepsy is a condition that affects the brain. When someone has epilepsy, it means they have a tendency to have epileptic seizures.

Anyone can have a one-off seizure, but this doesn't always mean they have epilepsy. Epilepsy is usually only diagnosed if someone has had more than one seizure, and doctors think it is likely they could have more.

Epilepsy can start at any age and there are many different types. Some types of epilepsy last for a limited time and the person eventually stops having seizures. But for many people epilepsy is a life-long condition.

WHAT ARE EPILEPTIC SEIZURES?

A seizure happens when there is a sudden burst of intense electrical activity in the brain. This causes a temporary disruption to the way the brain normally works.

The result is an epileptic seizure.

There are many different types of seizure. What happens to someone during a seizure depends on which part of their brain is affected. During some types of seizure, the person may remain alert and aware of what's going on around them, and with other types they may lose awareness. They may have unusual sensations, feelings, or movements. Or they may go stiff, fall to the floor and jerk.

WHAT CAUSES EPILEPSY?

Possible causes of epilepsy include:

- **Stroke**
- **A brain infection, such as meningitis**
- **Severe head injury**
- **Problems during birth which caused the baby to get less oxygen**

But in over half of all people with epilepsy, doctors don't know what caused it. Some may have a family history of epilepsy, suggesting that they may have inherited it.

Tonic-clonic seizures are the type of seizure most people recognise.

Someone having a tonic-clonic seizure goes stiff, loses responsiveness, falls to the floor and begins to jerk or convulse. They may go blue around the mouth due to irregular breathing. Sometimes they may lose control of their bladder or bowels, and bite their tongue or the inside of their mouth.

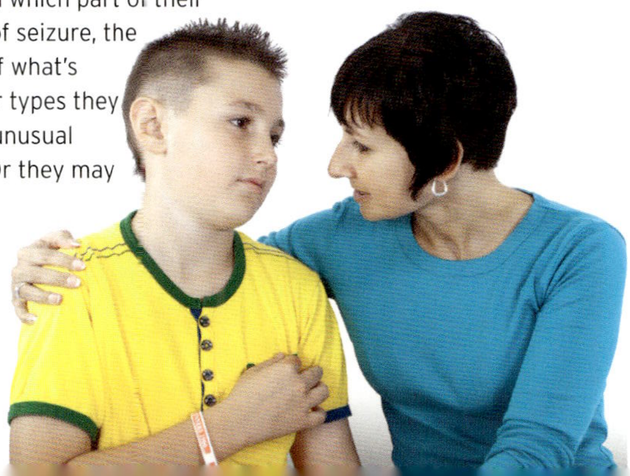

HOW TO HELP IF YOU SEE SOMEONE HAVING A TONIC-CLONIC SEIZURE

Do:

- **Protect them from injury (remove harmful objects from nearby)**
- **Cushion their head**
- **Look for an epilepsy identity card or identity jewellery - it may give you information about their seizures and what to do**
- **Time how long the jerking lasts**
- **Aid breathing by gently placing them in the recovery position once the jerking has stopped**
- **Stay with the them until they are fully recovered**
- **Be calmly reassuring**

Don't:

- **Restrain their movements**
- **Put anything in their mouth**
- **Try to move them unless they are in danger**
- **Give them anything to eat or drink until they are fully recovered**
- **Attempt to bring them round**

Call for an ambulance if:

- **You know it is their first seizure or**
- **The jerking continues for more than five minutes or**
- **They have one tonic-clonic seizure after another without regaining responsiveness between seizures or**
- **They are injured during the seizure or**
- **You believe they need urgent medical attention**

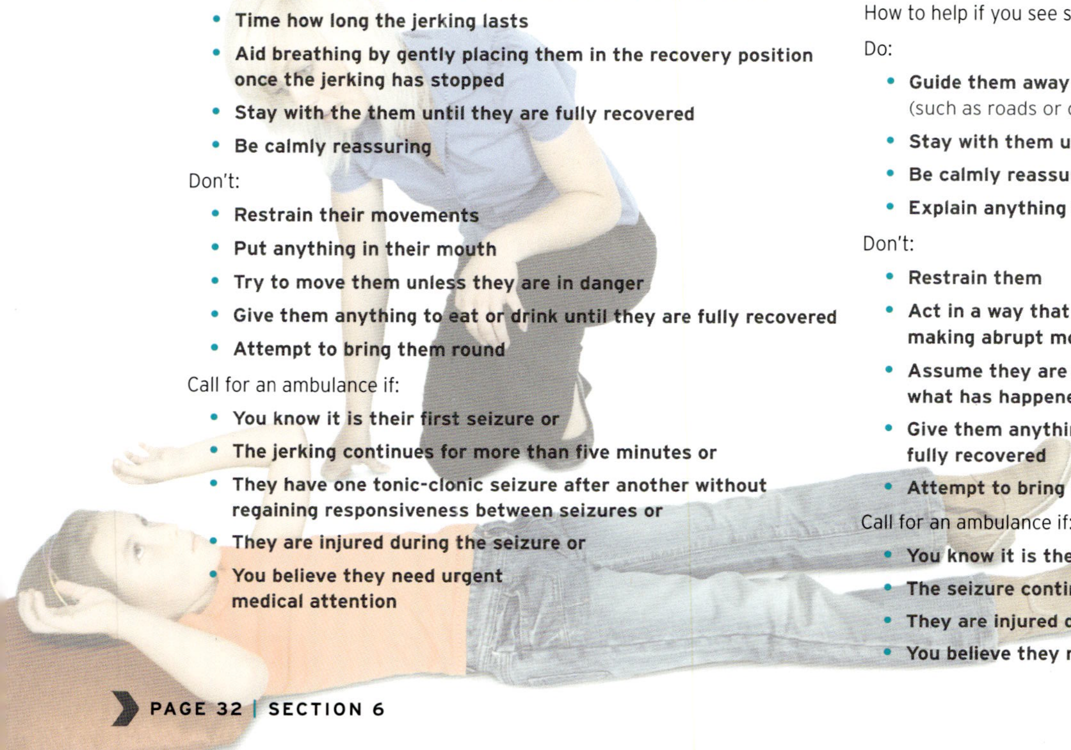

FOCAL SEIZURES

This type of seizure can also be called a partial seizure. Someone having a focal seizure may not be aware of their surroundings or what they are doing. They may have unusual movements and behaviour such as plucking at their clothes, smacking their lips, swallowing repeatedly or wandering around.

How to help if you see someone having a focal seizure.

Do:

- **Guide them away from danger** (such as roads or open water)
- **Stay with them until recovery is complete**
- **Be calmly reassuring**
- **Explain anything that they may have missed**

Don't:

- **Restrain them**
- **Act in a way that could frighten them, such as making abrupt movements or shouting at them**
- **Assume they are aware of what is happening, or what has happened**
- **Give them anything to eat or drink until they are fully recovered**
- **Attempt to bring them round**

Call for an ambulance if:

- **You know it is their first seizure or**
- **The seizure continues for more than five minutes or**
- **They are injured during the seizure or**
- **You believe they need urgent medical attention**

AIRWAY OBSTRUCTION

When a foreign body enters the airway the child reacts immediately by coughing in an attempt to expel it
A spontaneous cough is likely to be more effective and safer than any manoeuvre you might perform. However, if coughing is absent or ineffective, and the object completely obstructs the airway, the child will become asphyxiated rapidly. Active interventions to relieve choking are therefore required only when coughing becomes ineffective, but they then must be commenced rapidly and confidently.

The majority of choking events in children occur during play or whilst eating, when a carer is usually present. Events are therefore frequently witnessed, and interventions are usually initiated when the child is responsive.

Choking is characterised by the sudden onset of respiratory distress associated with coughing, gagging, or stridor, a high-pitched wheeze. Similar signs and symptoms may also be associated with other causes of airway obstruction, such as laryngitis or epiglottitis, which require different management.

Suspect choking caused by a foreign body if:

- **The onset was very sudden**
- **There are no other signs of illness**
- **There are clues to alert you, for example a history of eating or playing with small items immediately prior to the onset of symptoms**

General signs of choking

- **Witnessed episode**
- **Coughing or choking**
- **Sudden onset**
- **Recent history of playing with or eating small objects**

Ineffective coughing

- **Unable to vocalise**
- **Quiet or silent cough**
- **Unable to breathe**
- **Cyanosis**
- **Decreasing level of responsiveness**

Effective cough

- **Crying or verbal response to questions**
- **Loud cough**
- **Able to take a breath before coughing**
- **Fully responsive**

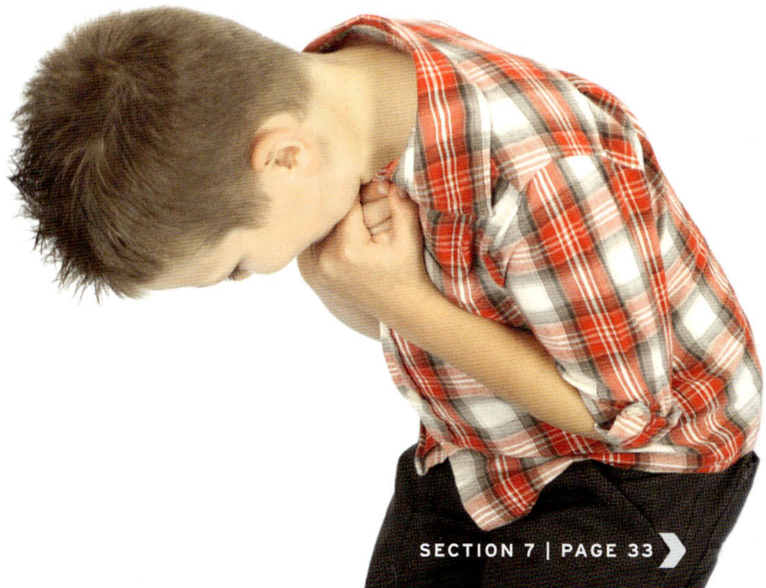

RELIEF OF CHOKING

Safety and summoning assistance

Safety is paramount. You should avoid placing yourself in danger and consider the safest action to manage the chcking child:

- **If the child is coughing effectively, then no external manoeuvre is necessary. Encourage the child to cough, and monitor continuously**
- **If the child's coughing is, or is becoming, ineffective, shout for help immediately and determine the child's responsive level**

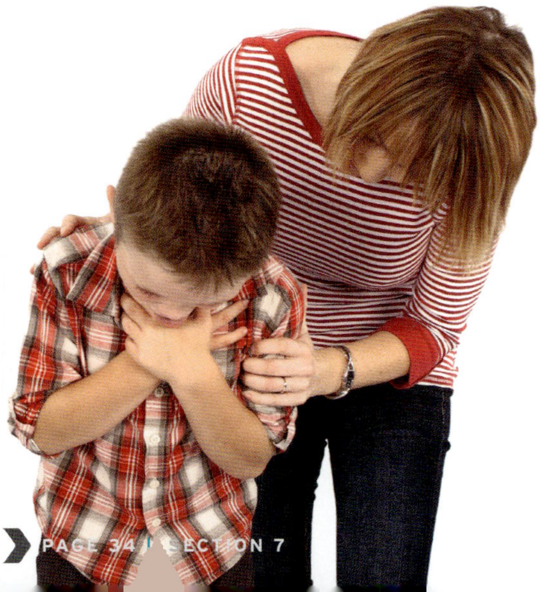

Responsive child who is choking

- **If the child is still responsive but has absent or ineffective coughing, give back blows**
- **If back blows do not relieve choking, give chest thrusts to infants or abdominal thrusts to children**

These manoeuvres create an 'artificial cough' to increase pressure in the chest cavity and dislodge the foreign body.

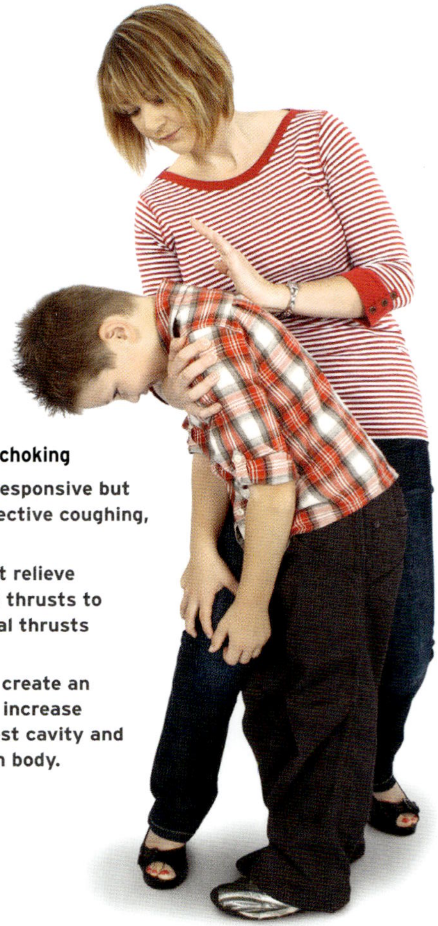

Back blows for an infant

- Support the infant in a head-downwards, prone position, to enable gravity to assist the removal of the foreign body
- If you are seated or kneeling, you should be able to support the infant safely across your lap

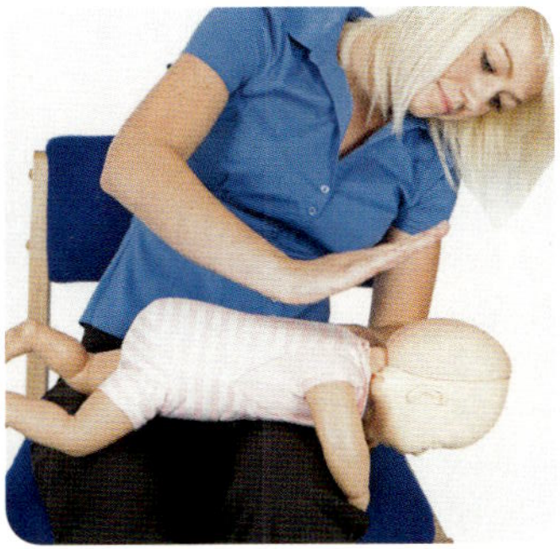

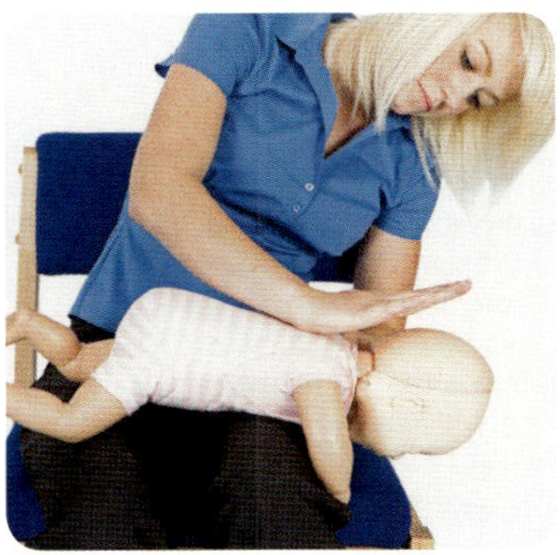

- Support the infant's head by placing the thumb of one hand at the angle of the lower jaw, and one or two fingers from the same hand at the same point on the other side of the jaw
- Do not compress the soft tissues under their jaw, as this will worsen the airway obstruction
- Deliver up to 5 sharp back blows with the heel of one hand in the middle of the back between the shoulder blades
- The aim is to relieve the obstruction with each blow rather than to give all 5

Back blows for a child

- Back blows are more effective if the child is positioned head down
- A small child may be placed across the rescuer's lap as with an infant

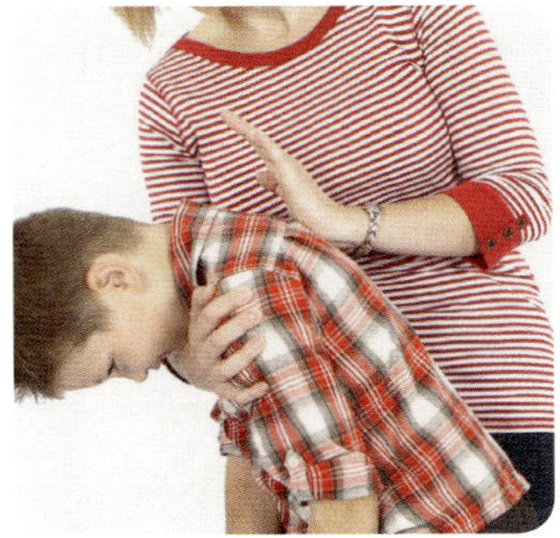

- If this is not possible, support the child in a forward-leaning position and deliver the back blows from behind

If back blows fail to dislodge the object, and they are still responsive, use chest thrusts for infants or abdominal thrusts for children. **Do not use abdominal thrusts for infants.**

Chest thrusts for infants:

- Turn them on to their back so they are facing up. With your free arm, support their head and ensure that the airway remains open without too much extension

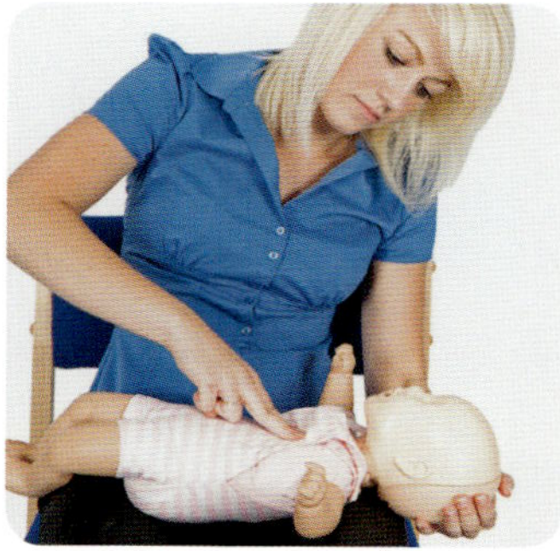

- Support them down your arm, which is placed down (or across) your thigh
- Identify the landmark for chest compression which is the centre of their chest on the lower part of their sternum
- Deliver up to 5 chest thrusts. These are similar to chest compressions, but sharper in nature and delivered at a slower rate
- The aim is to relieve the obstruction with each thrust rather than to give all 5

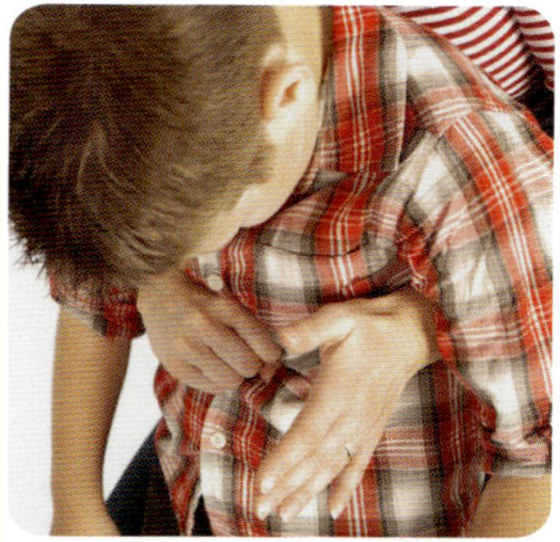

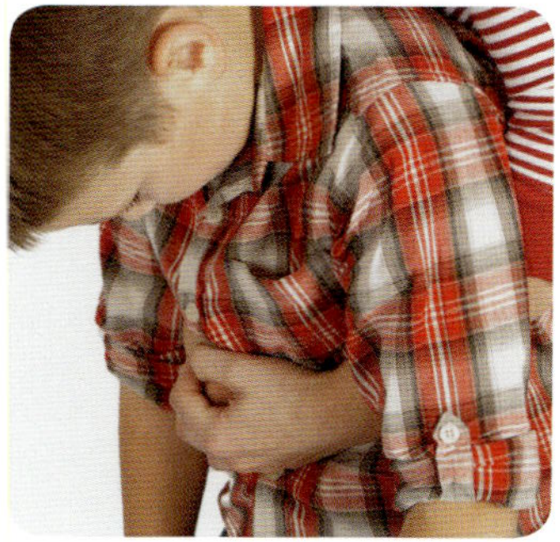

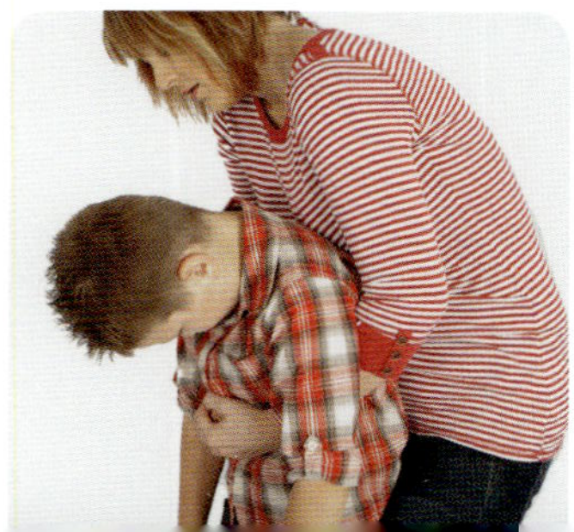

Abdominal thrusts for children over 1 year:

- Stand or kneel behind them and place your arms under their arms and encircle their torso
- Clench your fist and place it between the navel and the bottom of their breastbone
- Grasp this hand with your other hand and pull sharply inwards and upwards
- Repeat up to 4 more times
- The aim is to relieve the obstruction with each thrust rather than to give all 5

Repeat the sequence of up to 5 back blows followed by up to 5 chest thrusts for an infant, up to 5 abdominal thrusts for a child, until the obstruction is relieved or they become unresponsive.

NB: If the obstruction is still there after 1 cycle of back blows and abdominal/chest thrusts, you must summon an ambulance immediately. If you have to make this call yourself, then take the child/infant with you. Continue with your treatment of up to 5 back blows followed by up to 5 abdominal or chest thrusts.

If the object is expelled successfully you must seek medical advice, particularly if chest thrusts or abdominal thrusts have been given.

Unresponsive child or infant who is choking

- If the choking child is, or becomes, unresponsive place them on a firm, flat surface
- Call for an ambulance immediately. Send your bystander to make this call if you have one
- Do not leave the child or infant on their own if you have to make this call yourself

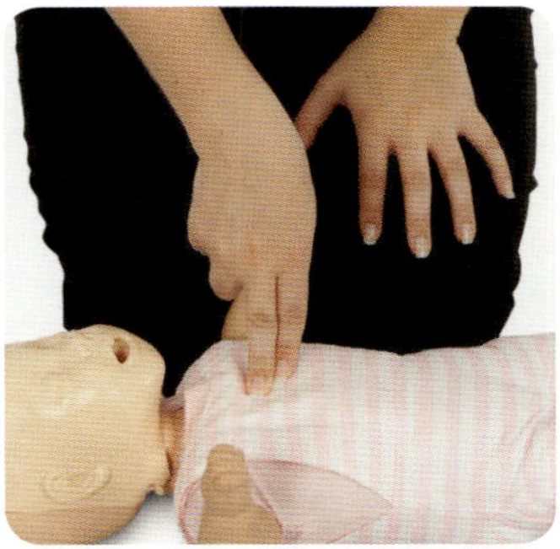

- Start CPR immediately (see page 20), but before each rescue breath attempt, look for any visible obstruction and remove it. If one is seen, make an attempt to remove it with a single finger sweep

Do not attempt blind or repeated finger sweeps
These can impact the object more deeply into the airway and cause injury.

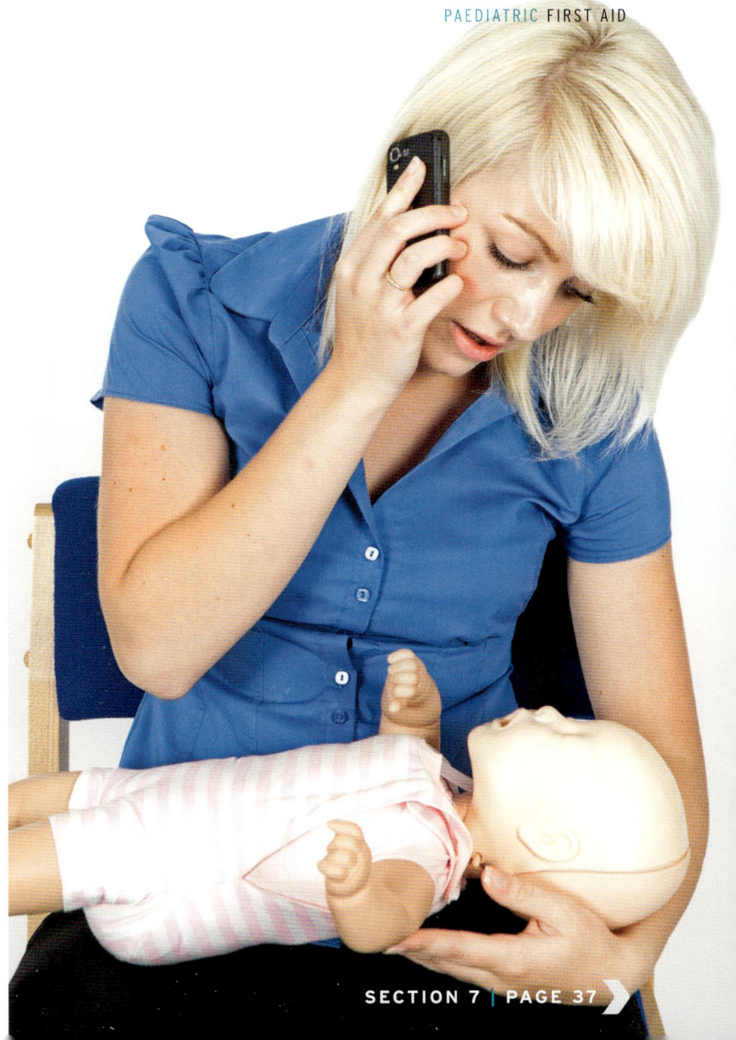

THE CIRCULATORY SYSTEM

The circulatory system is our body's transport system for two fluids, namely, blood and lymph.

For the purposes of First Aid we will focus on the transport of blood, also known as the cardio-vascular system.

This system consists of the heart and blood vessels, which supply our body, and in particular, our vital organs such as the brain and heart, with blood containing oxygen and nutrients to keep them healthy.

Our heart is a hollow muscular pump, about the size of your fist, with two pairs of chambers. These chambers collect blood flowing back from our body after depositing the oxygen and nutrients, before being pumped back to the lungs to collect more oxygen so that the cycle of transportation can continue.

The adult heart beats approximately 60 - 80 times every minute and pumps approximately six litres of blood around our body every minute.

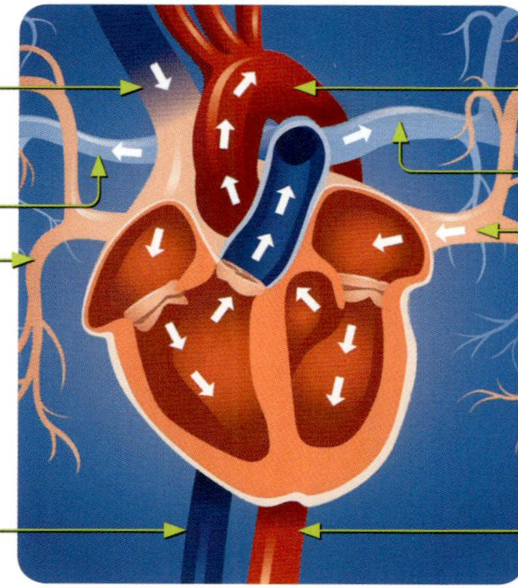

The blood vessels within this system are:

- **Arteries**
  Deliver oxygenated blood from the heart to the body, with the exception of the pulmonary artery which carries de-oxygenated blood from the heart to the lungs
- **Veins**
  Carry the de-oxygenated blood back to the heart
- **Capillaries**
  Much smaller vessels that form a link between the arteries, veins and body tissue to allow the transfer of oxygen and nutrients to the body and the waste products to be removed

Blood is made up of:

- **Plasma**
  The fluid component of the blood of which 90% is water
- **Platelets**
  Help to block the blood flow by clotting
- **Red cells**
  Transport the oxygen via the haemoglobin
- **White cells**
  Manufacture antibodies and fight infection and bacteria

There are a number of reasons why this system could fail, including blood loss, failure of the heart, poor circulation, a fall in blood pressure and the lack of oxygen contained within the body.

Other conditions include poisoning, vomiting, infection, burns and injury to the spinal cord, but this is by no means the definitive list.

As a First Aider, there are a number of things we can do for our casualty such as to stop the bleeding and to take pressure off the heart. This will be covered later, but one of your main concerns should be that hypovolaemic shock will set in very quickly if you don't react quickly enough, and shock can be a killer!

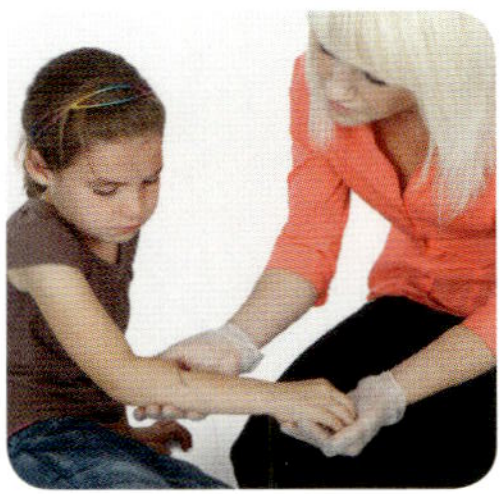

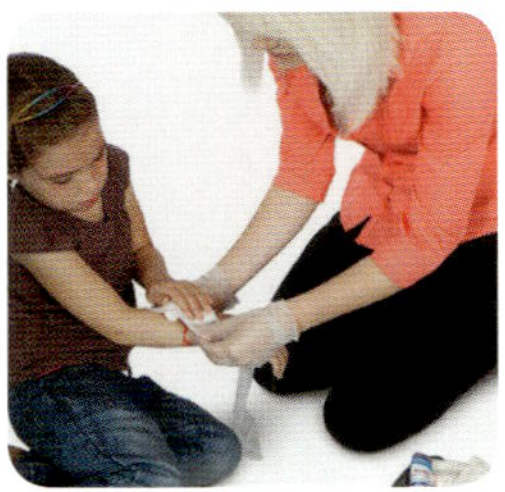

Hypovolaemic shock is best described as a failure or collapse of the circulatory system when the arterial blood pressure is too low to provide an adequate blood supply to the tissues.

Signs and symptoms of hypovolaemic shock

- **Ashen coloured skin (grey/blue)**
- **Clammy and cold skin to touch**
- **Feeling of sickness and thirst**
- **Their breathing will be rapid and shallow**

Treatment of hypovolaemic shock

- **Deal with the injury or condition**
- **Make them comfortable and lay them down**
- **Raise both legs providing it does not compromise their injuries further**
- **Keep them warm and maintain their response levels by talking to them**
- **Call for an ambulance**
- **Monitor their response and breathing**
- **Do not allow them to smoke, eat or drink as it may affect their well-being and it could compromise further treatment**

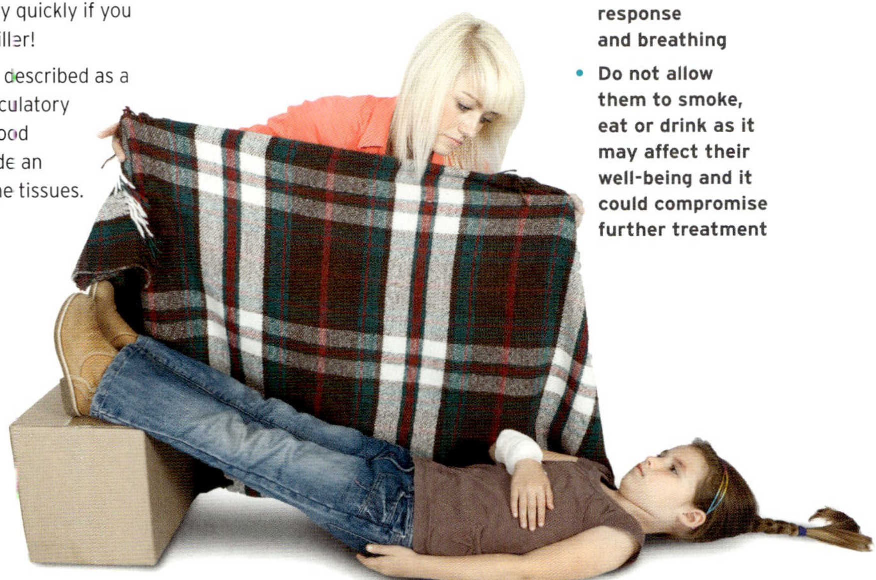

FAINTING

Fainting is a sudden, usually temporary, brief loss of responsiveness generally caused by insufficient oxygen in the brain.

The signs and symptoms are the same as shock with the exception that the pulse rate is slower.

A casualty who has fainted will generally make a rapid recovery and feel fine very quickly.

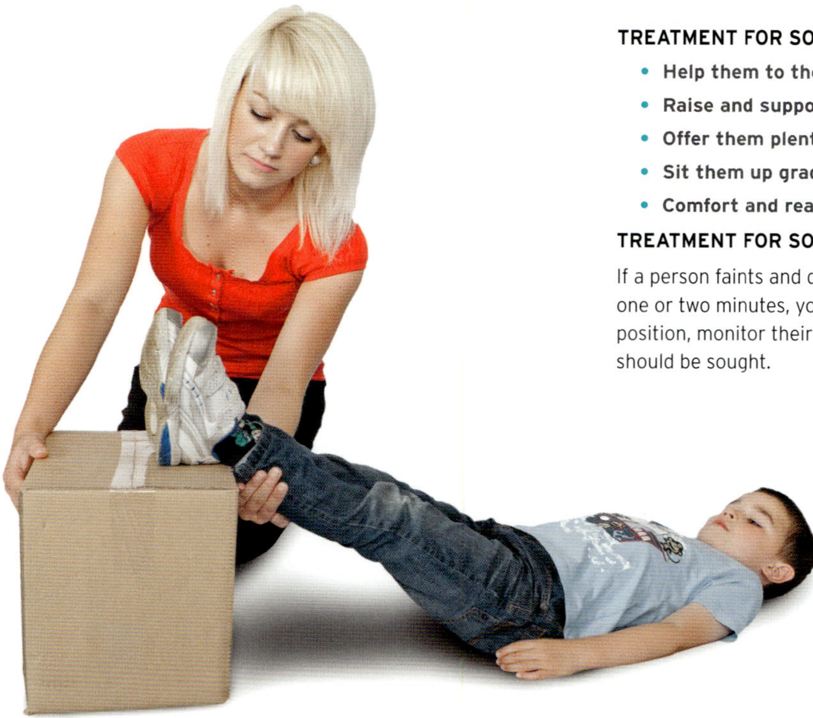

TREATMENT FOR SOMEONE WHO FEELS FAINT

- **Help them to the floor and lie them down**
- **Raise and support their legs**
- **Offer them plenty of fresh air**
- **Sit them up gradually**
- **Comfort and reassure them**

TREATMENT FOR SOMEONE WHO HAS FAINTED

If a person faints and does not regain responsiveness within one or two minutes, you should put them into the recovery position, monitor their breathing ,and medical assistance should be sought.

A wound can be best described as a type of injury in which the skin is torn, cut or punctured (an open wound), or where a blunt force created a contusion (a bruise).

In First Aid there are 6 types of wounds that you should be familiar with:

INCISION
Clean cut as with a knife blade

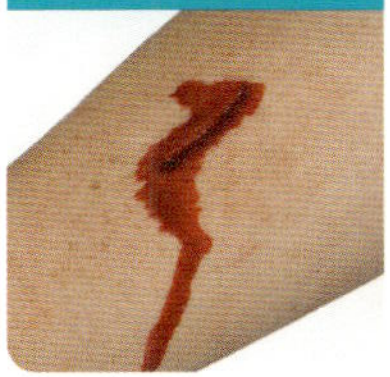

LACERATION
Rough tear as with barbed wire

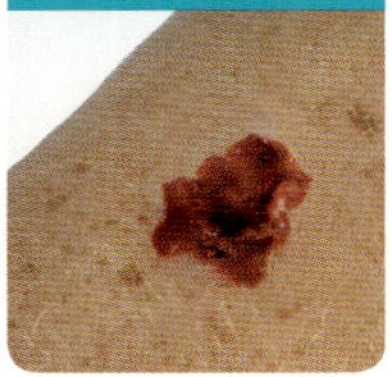

ABRASION
Scrape as with a gravel rash

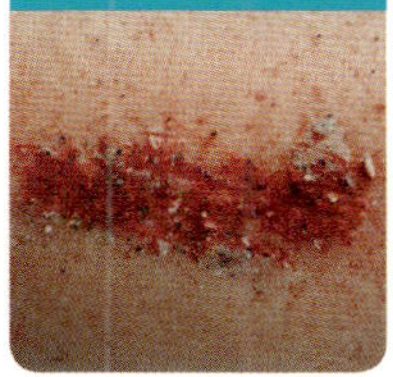

CONTUSION
A blunt blow causing bruising

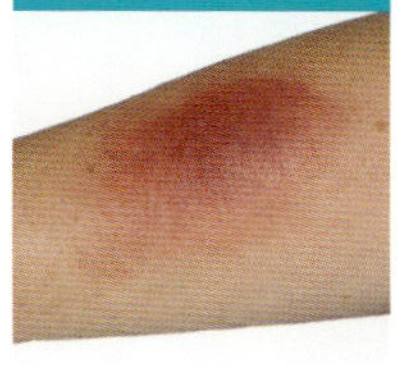

PUNCTURE
A stabbing type wound

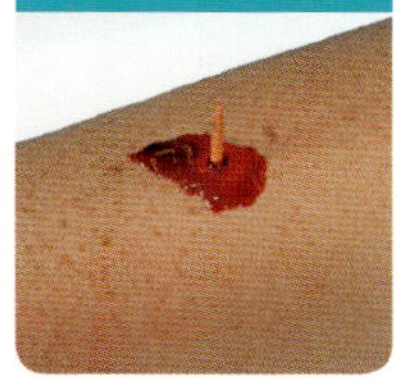

VELOCITY
Gunshot wound

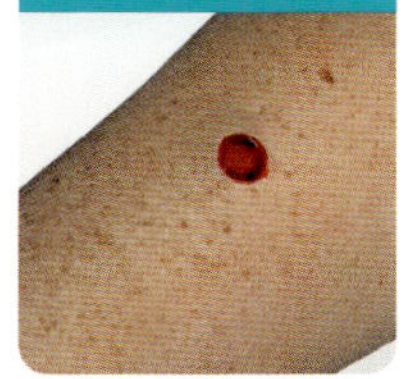

When a blood vessel is torn or severed, blood loss and shock cause the blood pressure to fall and the injured vessels will contract at the site of injury.

Platelets and proteins come into contact with the injured site and plug the wound.

This clotting process begins within ten minutes if the loss of blood is brought under control.

BLEEDING IS CLASSIFIED BY THE TYPE OF BLOOD VESSEL THAT IS DAMAGED.

Arterial Pumps from the wound with the heartbeat

Venous Gushes from the wound or pools at the site

Capillary Oozing at the site of injury

Once you have completed your initial casualty assessment for prioritising your treatment, you must follow the guidelines for personal protection and hygiene control before you begin to treat the casualty for bleeding (see page 42).

WOUNDS AND BLEEDING continued

Treatment for the control of bleeding

- **Put on disposable gloves**
- **Expose and examine the wound**
- **Apply direct pressure with your fingers or palm, preferably over a sterile dressing or non-fluffy clean pad (you can ask your casualty to apply this pressure)**
- **Elevate and support the injured part for wounds that are not catastrophic**
- **Help the casualty to lie down and raise the legs if you suspect shock**
- **Secure the dressing with a bandage large enough to cover the wound**
- **If further bleeding occurs, apply a second dressing on top of the first**
- **If blood seeps through this dressing, remove both dressings and apply a new one, making sure that pressure is applied accurately to the point of bleeding**
- **Support the injured limb with a sling or bandaging, providing the casualty allows you to do so**
- **Monitor their response levels and call for an ambulance**

CATASTROPHIC BLEEDING

If you are unable to stop the bleeding because of the severity, then you will need to apply direct pressure continually and then pack the wound with haemostatic dressings, or apply a tourniquet.

If you have neither, then you must continue to apply direct pressure and consider making an improvised tourniquet. It is imperative that you call for an ambulance immediately for a severe, or catastrophic bleed.

To summarise the treatment for catastrophic bleeding

- **Do apply direct pressure to the wound**
- **Do use a haemostatic dressing or tourniquet**
- **Do not apply indirect pressure to proximal pressure points**
- **Do not elevate an extremity**

Fortunately, the vast majority of businesses would never have to deal with a catastrophic bleed in a First Aid situation at work. For most First Aiders, blood loss can be controlled by following the guidelines as detailed to the left of this text.

It must be emphasised that further training is required for First Aiders in respect of using haemostatic dressings or tourniquets.

Please speak to your training provider.

EMBEDDED OBJECTS

If during your examination of the wound you see an embedded object such as a piece of glass, then you must leave it in place and dress around it.

Your aim is to stop the bleeding, but care must be taken not to put any direct pressure on the embedded object.

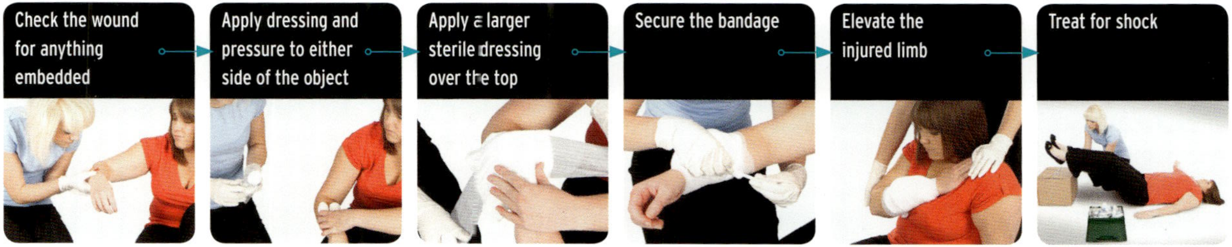

BLEEDING FROM ORIFICES

Signs, symptoms and causes

Site	Appearance	Cause
Mouth	Bright red, frothy, coughed up. Vomited blood, red or dark reddish brown.	Bleeding in the lungs. Bleeding in the stomach.
Ear	Fresh bright-red blood. Thin, watery blood.	Injury to ear, perforated eardrum. Head injury.
Nose	Fresh bright red blood. Thin, watery blood.	Ruptured blood vessel in nostril. Skull fracture.
Anus	Fresh bright-red blood. Black tarry, offensive smelling stool.	Injury to anus or lower bowel. Injury to upper bowel.
Urethra	Urine with red or smoky appearance and occasional clots.	Bleeding from the bladder, kidneys.
Vagina	Either fresh or dark blood	Menstruation, miscarriage, disease or injury to the vagina or womb.

TREATMENT

- **Treat the cause where possible using sterile dressings**
- **Treat the casualty for shock**
- **Monitor their condition, particularly their breathing**
- **Call 999/112 for an ambulance**
- **Lay them injured side down where possible**
- **Do not try to plug the wound, but cover it with a sterile dressing**
- **Offer them plenty of reassurance**
- **Pay attention to the casualty's modesty and dignity, particularly if they are bleeding from the anus or vagina**

AMPUTATIONS

Any part of the body that has been severed will need immediate hospital treatment.

There is almost certain to be severe blood loss, and your aim as an Emergency First Aider is to control the bleeding, treat for shock and to protect and transport the amputated body part to hospital with the casualty.

Your prompt and effective treatment may just allow the amputated part to be stitched back successfully with micro-surgery.

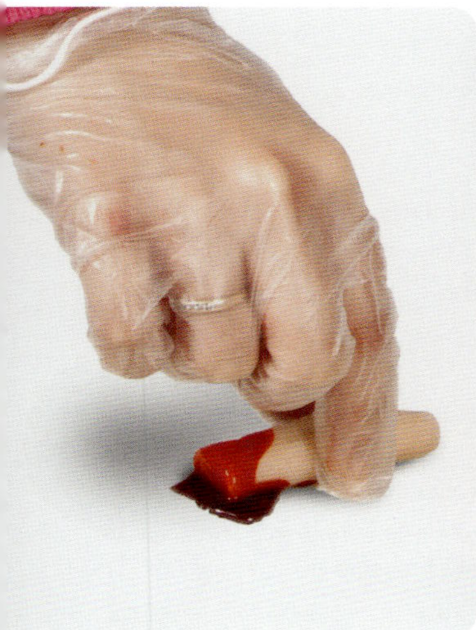

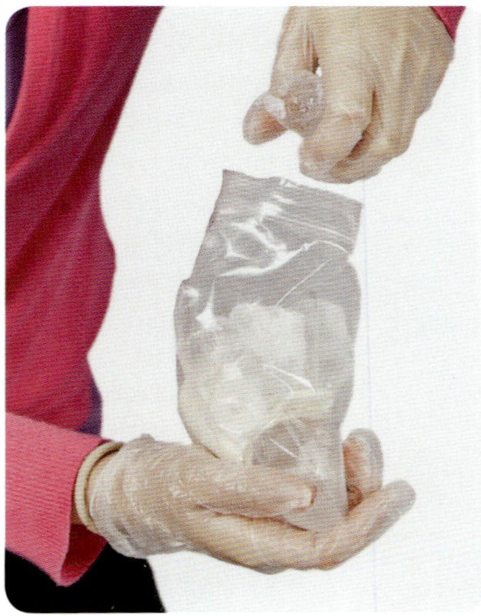

Signs and symptoms

- **Bleeding**
- **Shock**
- **Severe pain in the majority of cases**
- **An open wound**
- **Amputated body part**

Treatment

- **Ensure that the area is safe. Turn off machinery etc, that may have caused the accident**
- **Control the loss of blood by applying direct pressure with a sterile, non-fluffy dressing**
- **Treat the casualty for shock**
- **Reduce the risk of cross-infection by wearing gloves**
- **Call 999/112 for an ambulance**
- **Wrap the amputated part in plastic such as cling-film**
- **Wrap it further in a cloth**
- **Submerge the wrapped and protected part in ice. It is important that the severed part does not make direct contact with the ice. Mark the package clearly with the casualty's name and ensure that it is transported to hospital with the casualty**
- **Protect and maintain an open airway**
- **Monitor their breathing. Be prepared to resuscitate the casualty if they stop breathing normally**

MINOR CUTS AND GRAZES

Cuts and grazes are some of the most common injuries.

Minor cuts and grazes (where only the surface layer of skin is cut or scraped off) may bleed and feel slightly painful, but the affected area will normally scab over and heal quickly.

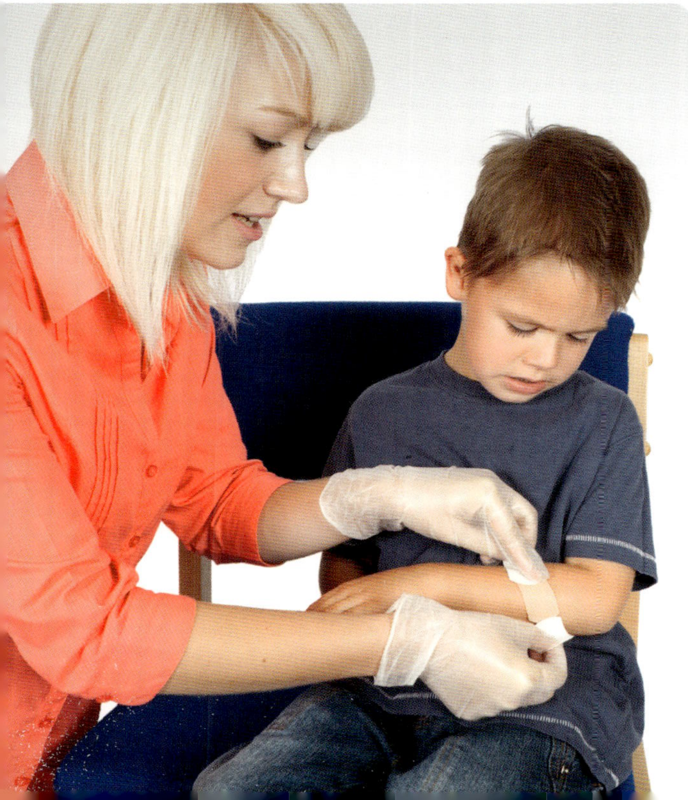

However, if the cut is in an area that is constantly moving, such as your knee joint, it may take longer to heal.

Depending on how deep the cut is and where it is on your body, a scar may remain once the cut has healed.

Deeper cuts may damage important structures below the skin such as nerves, blood vessels or tendons.

However, grazes that remove the deeper layers of skin are rare.

Most cuts and grazes can be easily treated by cleaning them thoroughly and covering them with a plaster or dressing.

Please bear in mind that hypoallergenic plasters are available should your casualty have an allergy to ordinary plasters.

SEEK MEDICAL HELP IF ANY OF THE BELOW APPLY:

You think there is damage to deeper tissues: signs include numbness (indicating injury to a nerve), blood spurting from the wound or bleeding that does not stop after five minutes of continuous firm pressure.

The wound is at risk of becoming infected: for example, a cut has been contaminated with soil, faeces or a dirty blade, or fragments of material such as grit or glass which can be seen in the wound.

The wound has become infected: signs include swelling of the affected area, pus coming from the wound, redness spreading from the wound and increasing pain. The wound cannot be closed with a plaster, or it starts to open up when it moves.

The wound will create an unwelcome scar: for example, if it occurs on a prominent part of the casualty's face.

BRUISING

Bruises are bluish or purple-coloured patches that appear on the skin when tiny blood vessels (capillaries) break or burst underneath it.

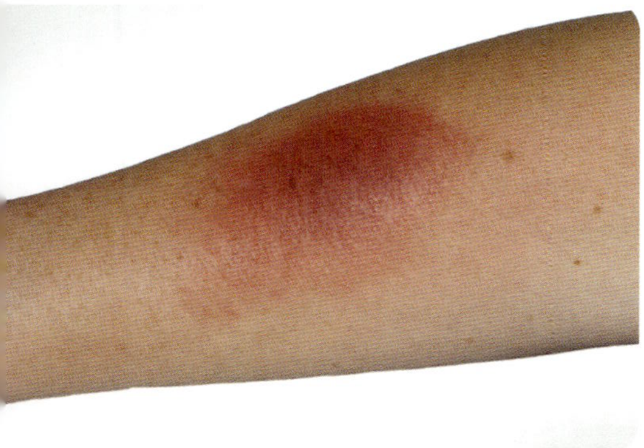

The blood from the capillaries leak into the soft tissue under the skin causing the discolouration.

Over time this fades through shades of yellow or green.

Bruises often feel tender or swollen at first.

WHAT CAUSES BRUISING?

Bruising is caused by internal bleeding (under the skin) due to a person injuring themselves by, for example, falling over, walking into something or playing sports.

Some people are naturally more likely to bruise than others, for example, the elderly may bruise more easily because their skin is thinner and the tissue underneath is more fragile.

Treatment for bruises

Treat bruises, initially, by limiting the bleeding. You can do this by cooling the area with a cold compress (a flannel or cloth soaked in cold water) or an ice pack wrapped in a towel.

To make an ice pack, place ice cubes or a packet of frozen vegetables in a plastic bag and wrap them in a towel. Hold this over the affected area for at least 10 minutes.

Do not put the ice pack straight onto the skin as this will possibly cause further damage.

Most bruises will disappear after around two weeks.

If the bruise is still there after two weeks, you should recommend that your casualty see their GP.

INTERNAL BRUISING

Bruises don't just happen under the skin - they can also happen deeper in the body's tissues, organs and bones.

While the bleeding isn't visible, the bruises can cause swelling and pain.

You should recommend that your casualty seeks medical attention, or call for an ambulance if you feel the injury is of a serious nature, particularly if they have been involved in an accident.

NOSE BLEEDS

A common injury that is caused generally by a direct blow or sneezing. However, high blood pressure can also cause a sudden bleed with little warning.

If the blood is watery, then it could suggest a head injury, therefore making the incident far more serious i.e. possible skull fracture.

Treatment

- **Sit the casualty down and lean them forward**
- **Ask them to pinch the soft part of the nose as they lean forward**
- **Apply this pressure for 10 minutes and then release slowly**
- **Ask them to avoid rubbing or blowing their nose**
- **If you are unable to stop the bleeding, ask them to repeat the pinching process for a further 10 minutes**
- **If the bleeding continues then you will need to seek medical advice**

If you suspect a head injury, then an ambulance must be summoned.

If the casualty is feeling faint or nausea you may consider sitting the casualty on the floor with their back supported. This could potentially prevent a fall.

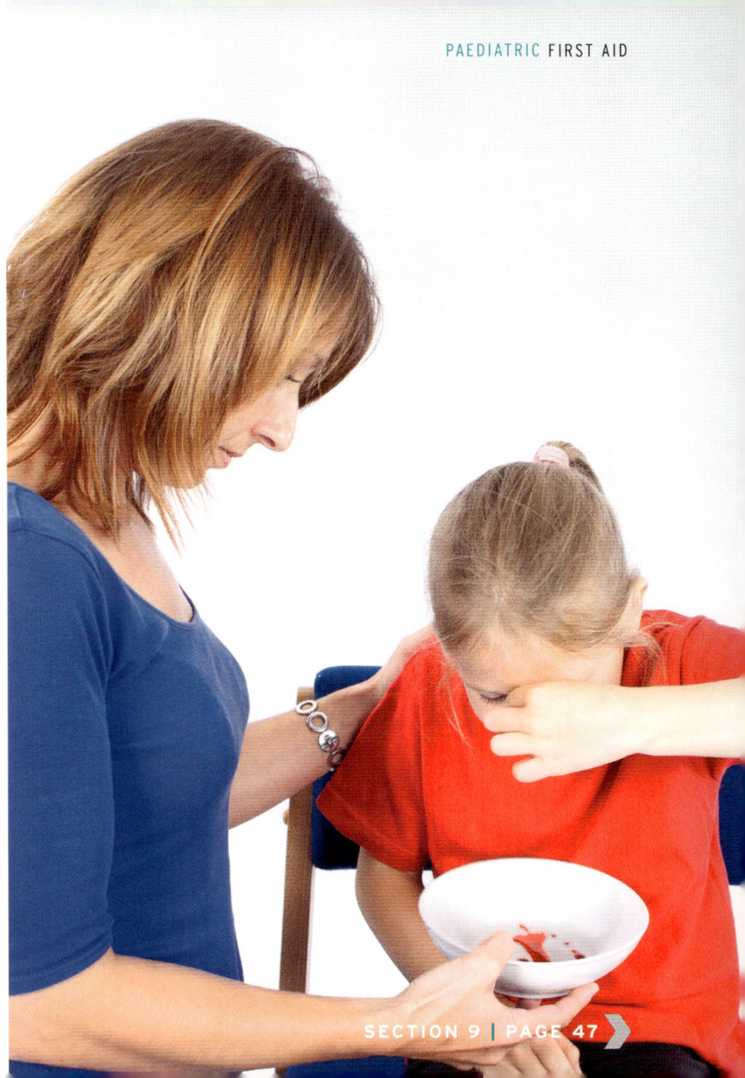

SMALL SPLINTERS

A foreign body or object in First Aid terms, relates to an object of any size that enters the body through many of its orifices, or penetrates the skin and is embedded.

You have to make a decision on whether you can remove it without having to seek medical help.

If a common embedded object such as a splinter is partly exposed, then it is acceptable to remove it with tweezers. First Aid tweezers generally come in a sterile package. Washing grit away, under running water, can also be a useful treatment. If this won't remove the object, then the wound should be dressed with a sterile dressing, without putting direct pressure on the object, and then to seek medical attention.

However, for other objects such as glass or a fishing hook, they must be left in place and you should not attempt to remove it. Dress the wound appropriately and seek medical advice.

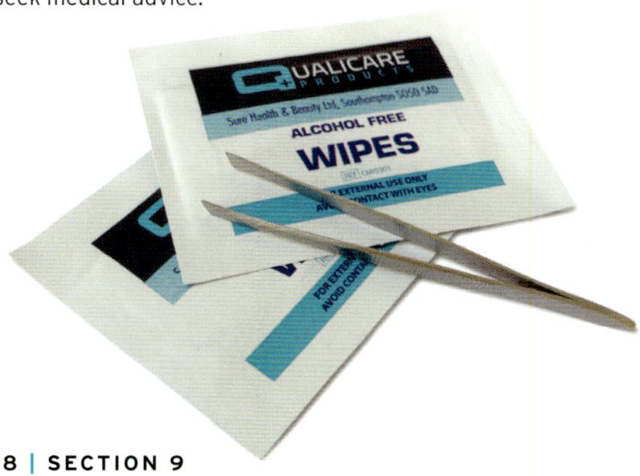

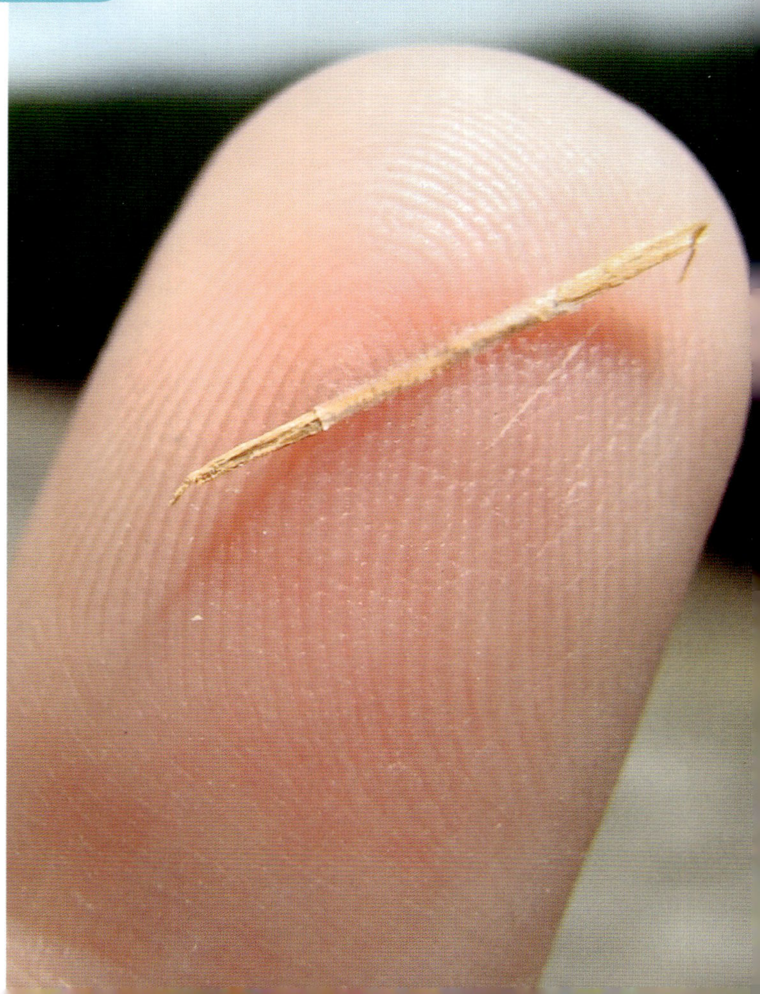

BITES AND STINGS

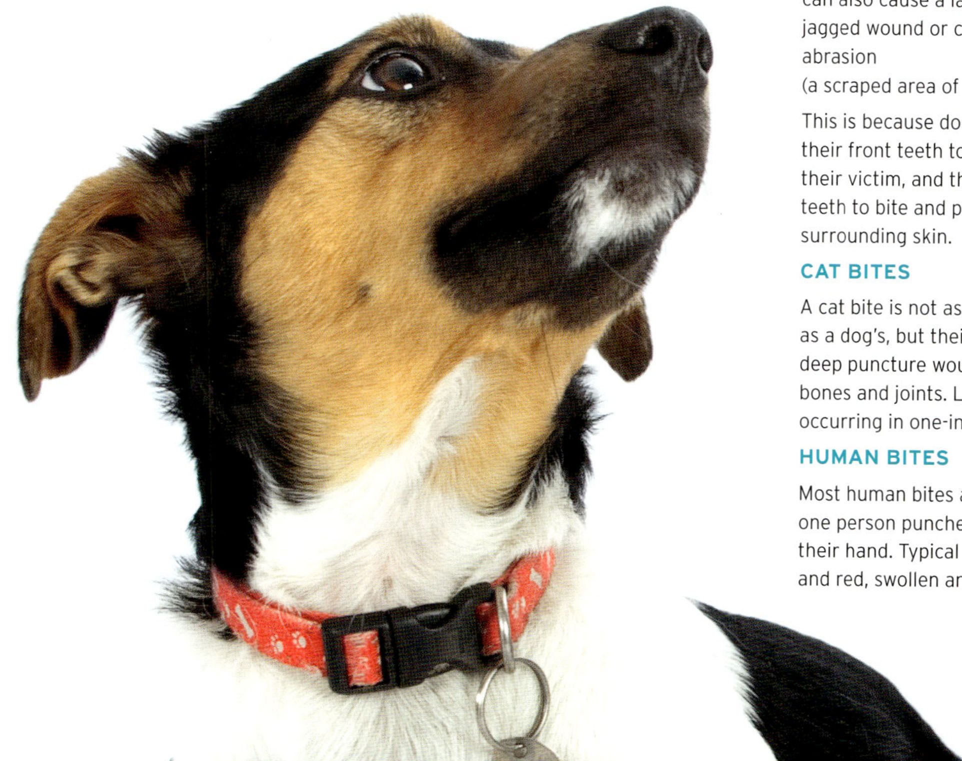

Animal and human bites are a relatively common type of injury. In most cases, the wound that results from an animal bite is minor and can be treated with simple First Aid techniques.

DOG BITES

Dog bites typically cause a puncture wound (a narrow and deep hole) in the skin. They can also cause a laceration (a jagged wound or cut) and an abrasion (a scraped area of skin).

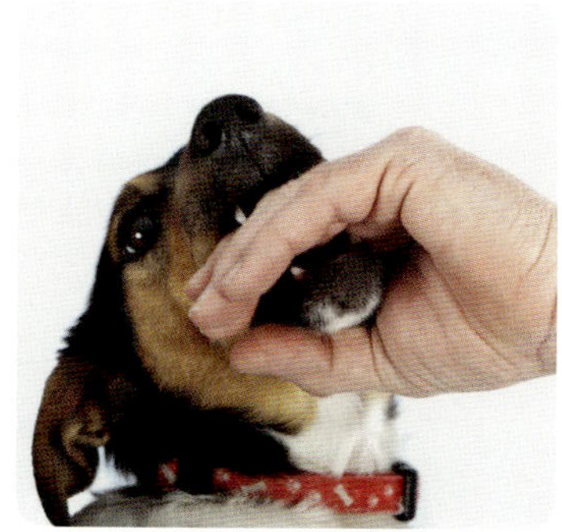

This is because dogs use their front teeth to "pin" their victim, and their other teeth to bite and pull at the surrounding skin.

CAT BITES

A cat bite is not as strong as a dog's, but their teeth are sharper and often cause very deep puncture wounds. A cat bite is capable of penetrating bones and joints. Lacerations and abrasions are less common, occurring in one-in-five cases.

HUMAN BITES

Most human bites are the result of a closed-fist injury, where one person punches another person in the teeth and cuts their hand. Typical symptoms include small cuts to the hand, and red, swollen and painful skin.

Toddlers often bite each other when playing together, but the resulting injuries are usually minor and do not usually pose a serious risk to their health.

General treatment

- **Make the area safe**
- **Reduce the risk of infection by wearing gloves**
- **Clean the wound immediately by running warm tap water over it for a couple of minutes**
- **Inspect the wound for embedded objects such as teeth and remove if you are able to**
- **Dry the wound and cover it with a sterile dressing**
- **Treat for shock**

When to seek medical advice:

You should seek immediate medical attention for all but minor dog or cat bites.

However, even some minor-looking cat bites can penetrate deeply and become infected.

Human bites have a much higher chance of causing infection, so always seek immediate medical attention before waiting for any symptoms of infection to appear.

Symptoms of infection

- **Redness and swelling around the wound. The wound becomes more painful**
- **Discharge from the wound**
- **Swollen lymph glands (nodes)**
- **A high temperature (fever) of 38°C (100.4°F) or above**
- **Shivers**

Always seek immediate medical attention if you or your child receives a bite to the following areas:

- **The hands**
- **The feet**
- **A joint, tendon or ligament**
- **The scalp or face**
- **The genitals**
- **The ears or nose**

Dial 999 immediately to request an ambulance if your child receives bite wounds to their head, neck or face. These types of wound can cause high amounts of blood loss, particularly in young children aged 10 or under and babies, and may therefore require emergency treatment.

If they have been bitten, the most important thing to do is to clean the wound immediately by running run warm tap water over the wound for 10 minutes.

In cases of serious bites, where a body part such as a finger or ear has been bitten off, you should wash the body part with tap water and place it in a plastic bag or a sealed container. Put the bag or container into a tub of iced water (but not frozen) to keep it cool, so that it can be transported to hospital. It may be possible to reattach the body part using reconstructive surgery.

Fortunately, in the seas around the UK, there are only a few types of marine creatures that sting.

These include weever fish, jellyfish, Portuguese man-of-war, sea urchins and stingrays. The symptoms and treatments for sea creature stings are all very similar. For the purposes of paediatric first aid, we will focus on weever fish and jellyfish.

WEEVER FISH

Weever fish have poisonous spines on their back and gills. Most people are stung on their feet by them after accidentally stepping on them.

Signs and symptoms

- **Severe pain**
- **Itching**
- **Swelling** (inflammation)
- **Redness**
- **Numbness**
- **Tingling**
- **Nausea**
- **Vomiting**
- **Headache**
- **Joint ache**
- **Abdominal cramps**
- **Lightheadedness**
- **Temors** (shaking)

If a person has a more serious reaction to a weever fish sting, they may experience:

- **An abnormal heart rhythm (arrhythmia)**
- **Shortness of breath**
- **Weakness**
- **Paralysis**
- **Seizures (fits)**
- **A drop in blood pressure**
- **Episodes of unresponsiveness**

Treatment

Seek medical assistance immediately.

To control the pain, the affected area should be immersed in hot water (as hot as can be tolerated) for between 30-90 minutes. This can be repeated if necessary. When the area has been numbed, be careful not to burn it with the hot water.

Thoroughly clean the wound using soap and water, before rinsing with fresh water. Do not cover the wound.

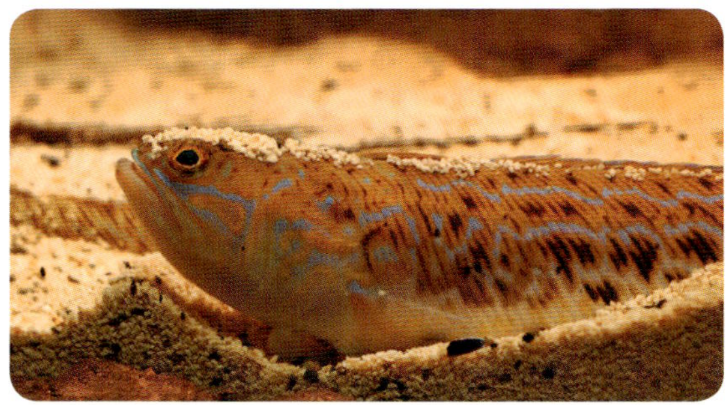

JELLYFISH

Jellyfish are mushroom-shaped creatures that have many long, thin tentacles on the underside of their bodies. The tentacles are covered with small poisonous sacs called nematocysts which, if touched, produce a nasty sting.

Jellyfish live in seas throughout the world and are found at a wide range of depths, although they often float near the surface. In recent years, during the warmer months, large swarms of jellyfish have become increasingly common in the seas around Europe, such as the Mediterranean.

Experts believe the increase in jellyfish numbers may be the result of increasingly warmer weather conditions combined with overfishing of their natural predators.

If you are stung by a jellyfish, you will experience some immediate symptoms such as:

- **Severe pain**
- **Itching**
- **A rash**
- **Raised welts (raised, circular areas on the skin)**

Other symptoms that you may have include:

- **Nausea**
- **Vomiting**
- **Diarrhoea**
- **Abdominal pain**
- **Muscle spasms**
- **Numbness**
- **Tingling**
- **Swollen lymph nodes**

(lymph nodes are small nodules that are found in several areas around the body, including in the groin and armpit)

In rare cases, a serious reaction to a jellyfish sting can result in breathing difficulties, coma or death.

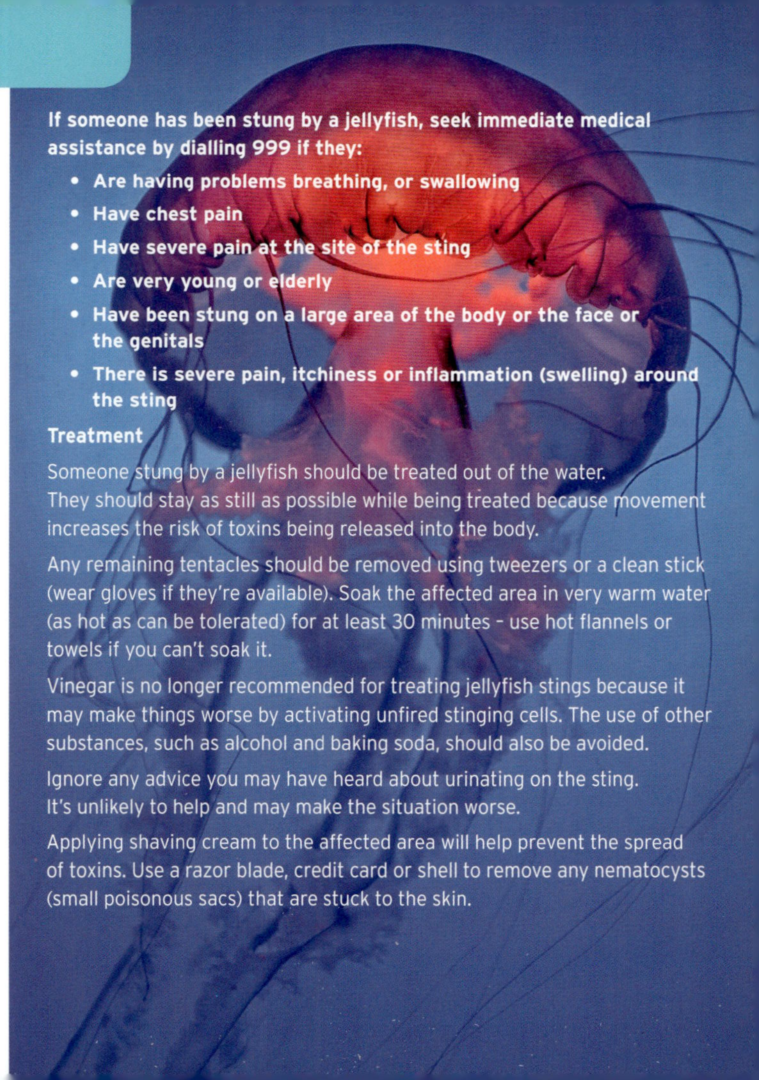

If someone has been stung by a jellyfish, seek immediate medical assistance by dialling 999 if they:

- **Are having problems breathing, or swallowing**
- **Have chest pain**
- **Have severe pain at the site of the sting**
- **Are very young or elderly**
- **Have been stung on a large area of the body or the face or the genitals**
- **There is severe pain, itchiness or inflammation (swelling) around the sting**

Treatment

Someone stung by a jellyfish should be treated out of the water. They should stay as still as possible while being treated because movement increases the risk of toxins being released into the body.

Any remaining tentacles should be removed using tweezers or a clean stick (wear gloves if they're available). Soak the affected area in very warm water (as hot as can be tolerated) for at least 30 minutes - use hot flannels or towels if you can't soak it.

Vinegar is no longer recommended for treating jellyfish stings because it may make things worse by activating unfired stinging cells. The use of other substances, such as alcohol and baking soda, should also be avoided.

Ignore any advice you may have heard about urinating on the sting. It's unlikely to help and may make the situation worse.

Applying shaving cream to the affected area will help prevent the spread of toxins. Use a razor blade, credit card or shell to remove any nematocysts (small poisonous sacs) that are stuck to the skin.

Many insects sting as a defence mechanism by injecting venom into the skin. In the UK, stinging insects include:

- **Bees** (honeybees and bumblebees)
- **Wasps**
- **Hornets**

Insect stings usually cause a swollen, red, raised mark to form on the skin. This is known as a weal. The affected area will often be painful and itchy. This will usually last for a few days.

If you are stung by an insect, such as a wasp, the area around the sting will become inflamed (swollen), go red and a raised mark (weal) will form. The affected area will often be quite painful and itchy. This will usually last for a few days.

People who have an allergic reaction to an insect sting will experience more symptoms. An allergic reaction occurs when the venom from the sting triggers the release of chemicals in the body, such as histamine.

Seek emergency medical treatment if, immediately after being stung, you experience any of the following:

- **Swelling or itching anywhere else on your body**
- **A skin reaction anywhere else, particularly pale or flushed (red or blotchy) skin**
- **Wheezing, hoarseness or any difficulty breathing**
- **A headache**
- **Nausea, vomiting or diarrhoea**
- **A fast heart rate**
- **Dizziness or feeling faint**
- **Difficulty swallowing (dysphagia)**
- **A swollen face or mouth**
- **Confusion, anxiety or agitation**

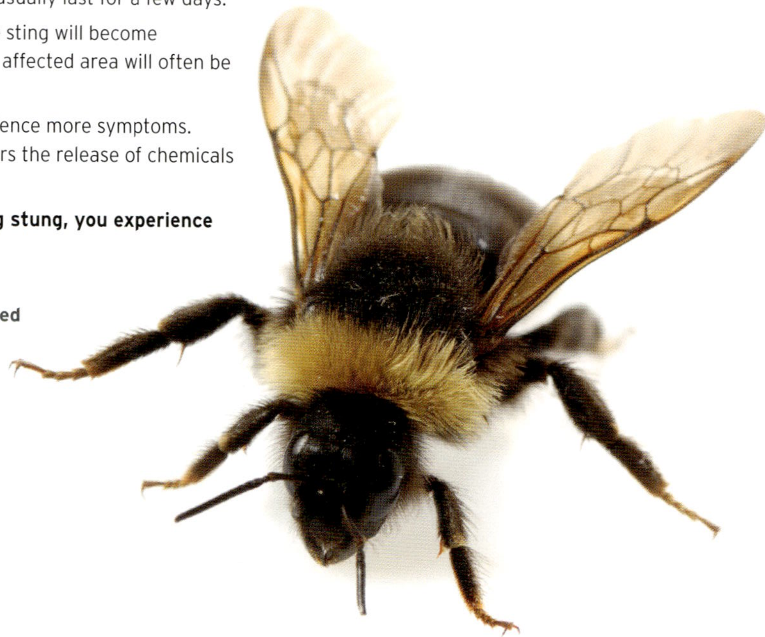

BITES AND STINGS continued

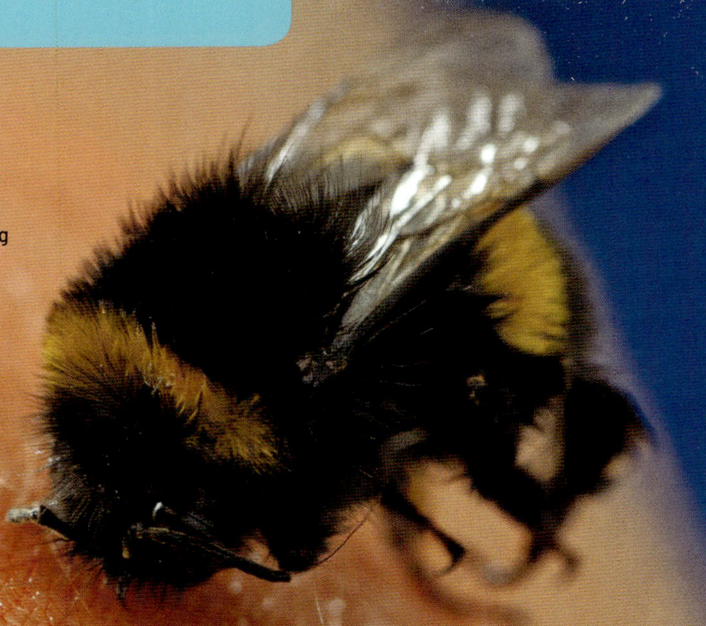

Treatment

Bee stings have a venomous sac attached. After you have been stung, the sting and the venomous sac will remain behind and the bee will die.

Wasps and hornets do not usually leave the sting behind and therefore could continue to sting you. If you have been stung and the wasp or hornet remains in the area, walk away calmly to avoid getting stung again.

Remove the sting immediately

As soon as you have been stung by an insect, you should remove the sting and the venomous sac. Do this by scraping it out with a hard edge, such as a bank card.

When removing the sting, be careful not to spread the venom further under your skin and that you do not puncture the venomous sac. Do not attempt to pinch the sting out with your fingers or a pair of tweezers, as you may spread the venom. If a child has been stung, an adult should remove the sting.

Basic treatment

To treat insect stings:

- **Wash the affected area with soap and water**
- **Put a cold flannel on the area**
- **Raise the part of the body that has been stung to prevent swelling**
- **Avoid scratching the area because it may become infected (see below)**
- **Keep children's fingernails short and clean**
- **Visit your GP if the redness and itching gets worse or does not clear up after a few days**

Snake bites

Snakes sometimes bite in self-defence if they are disturbed or provoked.

Adders, or vipers, are the only wild venomous snakes in the UK.

Adders sometimes bite without injecting any venom (toxins produced by the snake).

This is called a 'dry' bite and may cause:

Mild pain caused by the adder's teeth puncturing the skin, and anxiety.

If an adder injects venom when it bites it can cause more serious symptoms including:

- **Swelling and redness in the area of the bite**
- **Nausea (feeling sick)**
- **Vomiting**
- **Faintness**

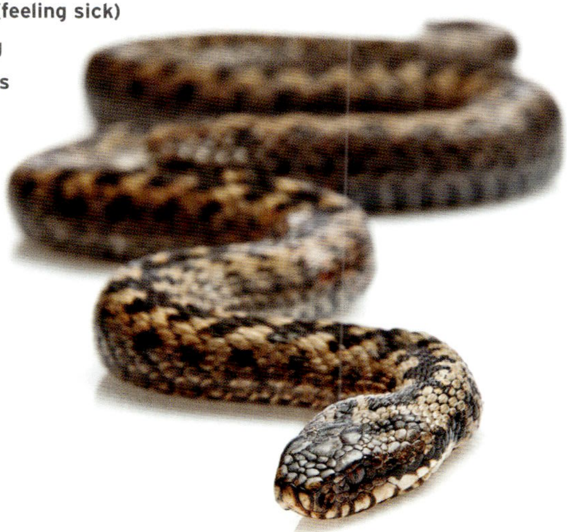

Immediate action

If a snake bites you, or someone else, you should follow the advice listed below.

- **Remain calm and do not panic. Snake bites, particularly those that occur in the UK, are rarely serious and very rarely fatal**
- **Try to remember the shape, size and colour of the snake**
- **Keep the part of your body that has been bitten as still as possible because this will prevent the venom spreading around your body. You may want to secure the bitten body part with a sling (a supportive bandage) or a splint (a rigid support that helps keep the body part stable). However, do not make the sling or splint so tight that it restricts your blood flow**
- **Remove any jewellery and watches from the bitten limb because they could cut into your skin if the limb swells. However, do not attempt to remove any clothing, such as trousers**
- **Seek immediate medical attention immediately**

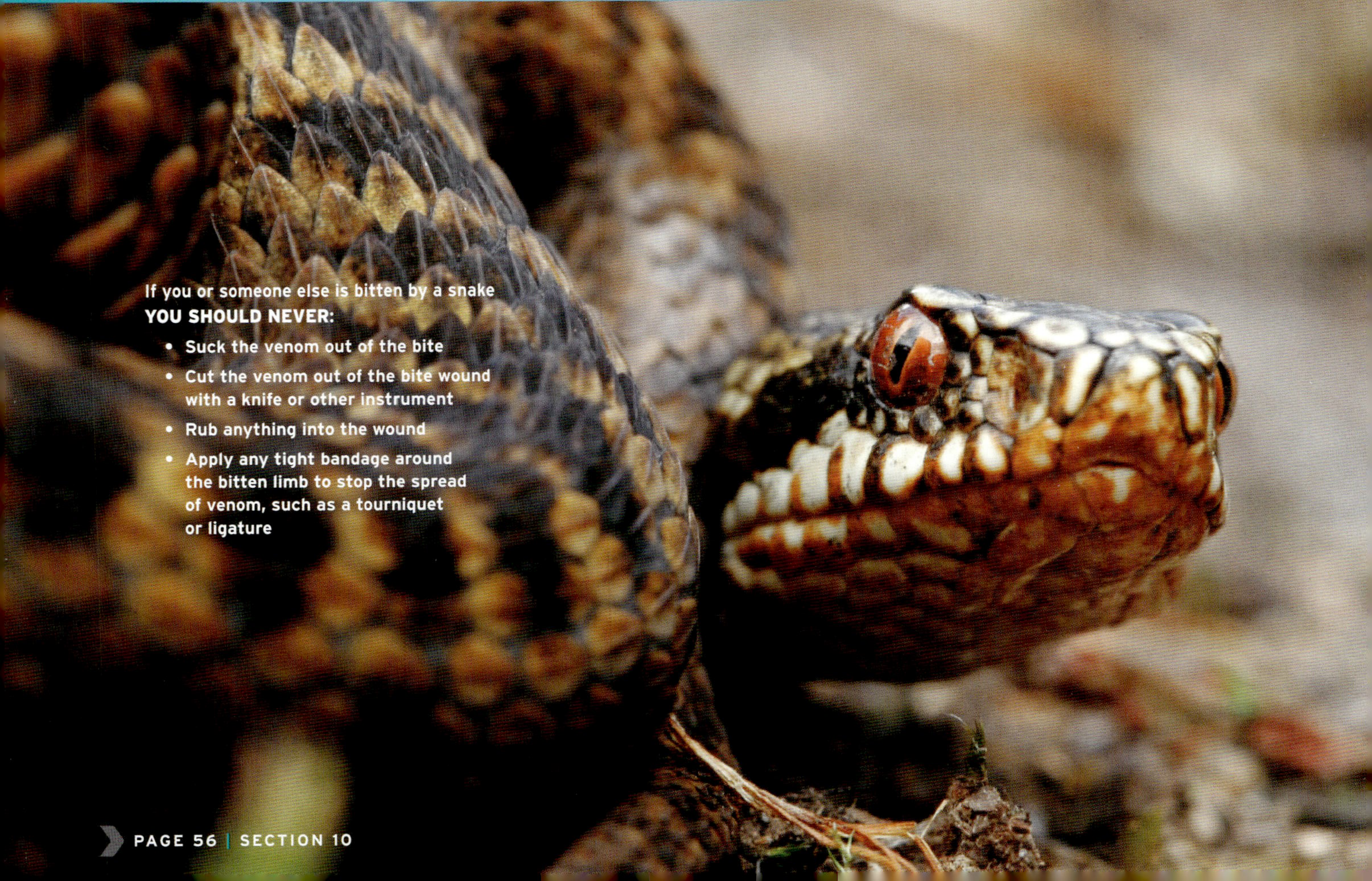

If you or someone else is bitten by a snake
YOU SHOULD NEVER:

- Suck the venom out of the bite
- Cut the venom out of the bite wound with a knife or other instrument
- Rub anything into the wound
- Apply any tight bandage around the bitten limb to stop the spread of venom, such as a tourniquet or ligature

PAEDIATRIC BASIC LIFE SUPPORT

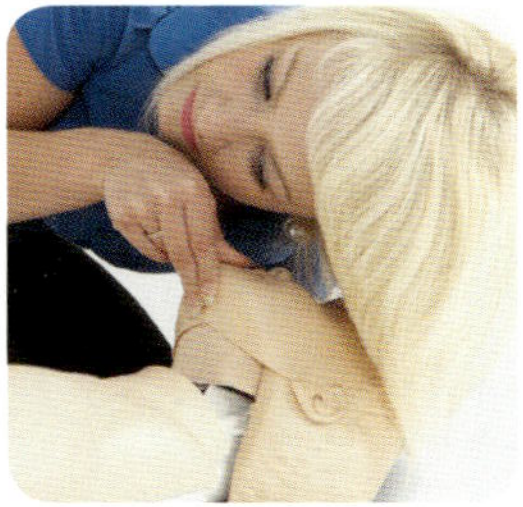

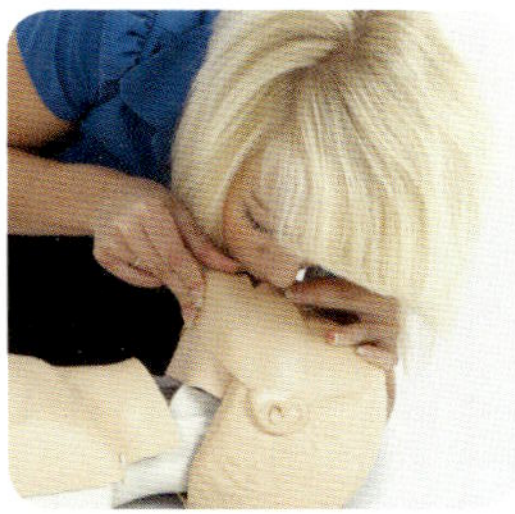

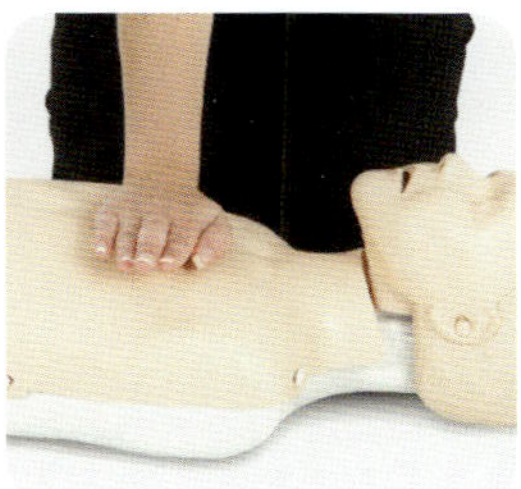

CHECK FOR DANGERS

CHECK FOR RESPONSE

YES → If responsive, check for injuries and treat accordingly. Call the emergency services if required.

NO → If you are on your own, you should shout for help.

OPEN THE AIRWAY → Use minimum head tilt and lift the chin carefully.

Check for normal breathing for no more than 10 seconds.

YES → If breathing normally, check for any injuries and place them in the recovery position. Call the emergency services and monitor their breathing.

NO

Give 5 initial breaths followed by 1 minute of CPR

If help is available, send them to call the emergency services and to bring a defibrillator back with them if one is available.

NO → If no help is available you must call them yourself and return with a defibrillator if one is available.

Continue with CPR until the casualty recovers, the emergency services take over or you become exhausted.

NB: If a defibrillator is available, then connect it immediately to the casualty and follow the voice prompts. If you have trained help available, then they can start CPR whilst you are preparing the casualty for defibrillation. (If you have access to an AED - See pages 25-29)

BONES, JOINTS AND MUSCLE INJURIES

The human skeleton is made up of 206 bones, the largest being the femur, or thigh bone.

It serves many purposes:

- **It protects vital organs such as the brain, heart and lungs**
- **It supports muscles held to the skeleton by tendons**
- **It provides movement in the form of joints which are held together by ligaments**

There are three types of joints:

1. **Non-movable - such as the bones that make up the skull**
2. **Partially movable - such as the ribs and spine**
3. **Movable joints - such as the hip, which is made up of a ball and socket**

Through various activities, bones can be damaged or broken.

Breaks or fractures fall into three main categories:

1. **Closed fracture. This is where the break does not penetrate the skin**
2. **Open fracture. This is where the broken bone does penetrate the skin**
3. **Complicated fracture. This is where the broken bone injures another part of the body i.e. a broken rib penetrating a lung**

In respect of First Aid, there is nothing you can do to repair the fracture. However, you can offer treatment that will make the casualty more comfortable in order to prevent the injury from worsening.

DO NOT attempt to straighten or realign a fracture.

Your aims are to:

- **Prevent movement of the broken bone**
- **Support them in the position found**
- **Call 999 for the emergency services**
- **Limit their pain**
- **Reduce the chance of further injury**
- **Facilitate safe and prompt transport**

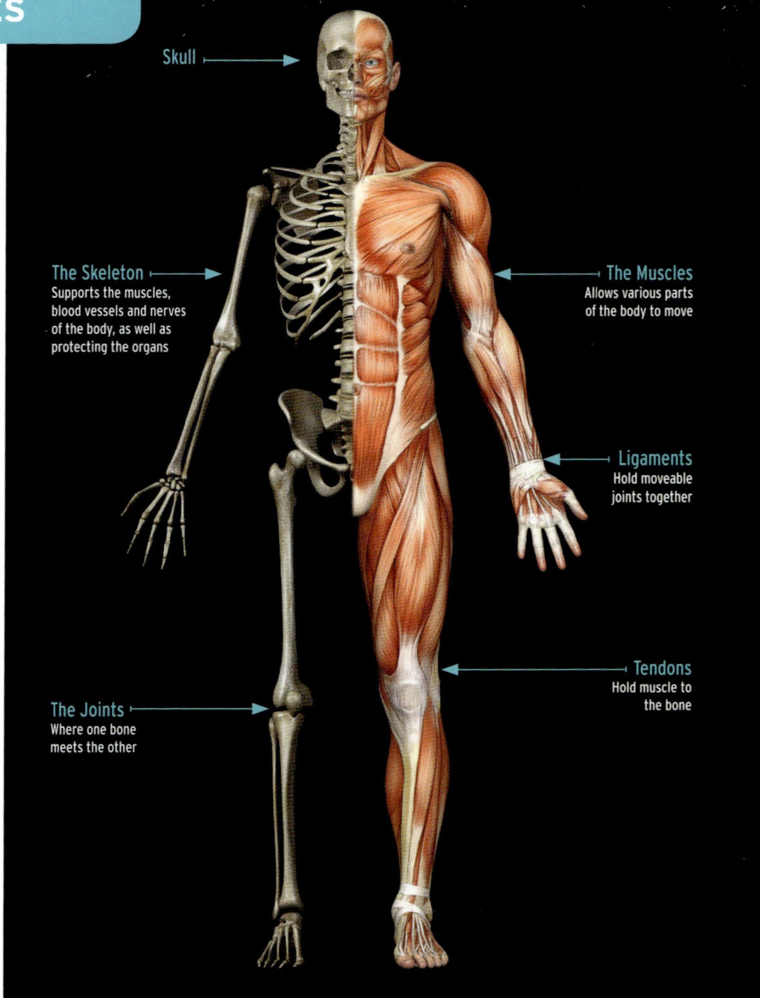

CLOSED FRACTURE

Signs and symptoms

- **Pain**
- **Swelling**
- **Deformity**
- **Internal bleeding**
- **Bruising**
- **Shock**

GREENSTICK FRACTURE

A greenstick fracture is a type of mild bone fracture which is most commonly seen in children. In this type of fracture, extreme force causes a bone to bend, breaking partway through, much like a green twig when it is bent.

This type of broken bone most commonly occurs in children because their bones are softer and more flexible than are the bones of adults.

The signs and symptoms will vary, depending on the severity of the greenstick fracture.

Mild fractures might be mistaken for sprains or bruises. More-severe greenstick fractures may cause an obvious deformity, accompanied by significant pain and swelling.

In respect of treatment, follow the guidelines as detailed on this page for a 'CLOSED FRACTURE'.

Treatment

- Immobilise the injured part to stop any movement
- Place padding around the injury for further support
- Leave the casualty in the position found unless they can move the injured part to a more comfortable position
- For additional support, particularly if there is a delay in the emergency services arriving, you could consider strapping an uninjured leg to the injured one. Use broad-fold bandages and ensure that any knots are tied to the uninjured side. Do not wrap a bandage over the fracture. If their circulation is impaired, loosen the dressings
- You MUST NOT try to realign the fracture. This should only be performed by medically trained professionals
- Do not give you casualty anything to eat or drink
- Treat for shock
- Call 999/112

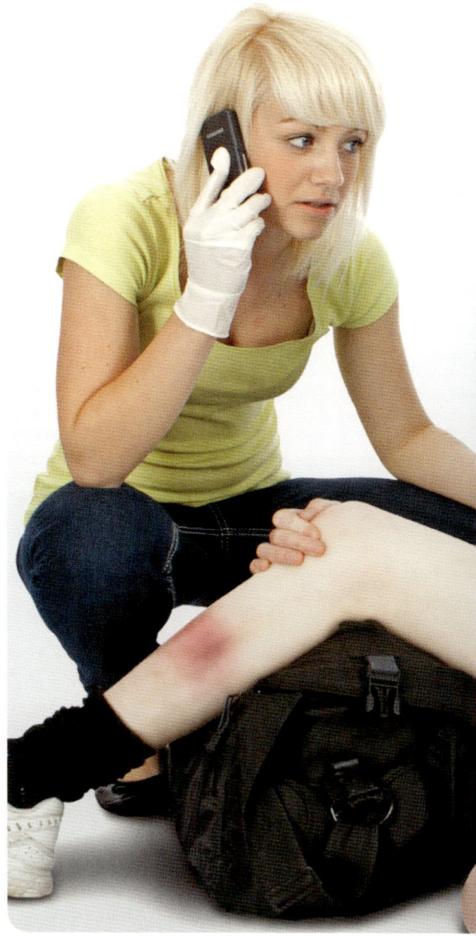

OPEN FRACTURE

Signs and symptoms

- Pain
- Deformity
- Internal bleeding
- External bleeding
- Shock

Treatment

- Call for an ambulance immediately
- Prevent any movement
- Reduce the risk of infection by wearing gloves
- Control the blood loss by dressing around the wound
- DO NOT apply any direct pressure on the protruding bone
- Use sterile non-fluffy dressings
- For additional support, particularly if there is a delay in the emergency services arriving, you could consider strapping an uninjured leg to the injured one.

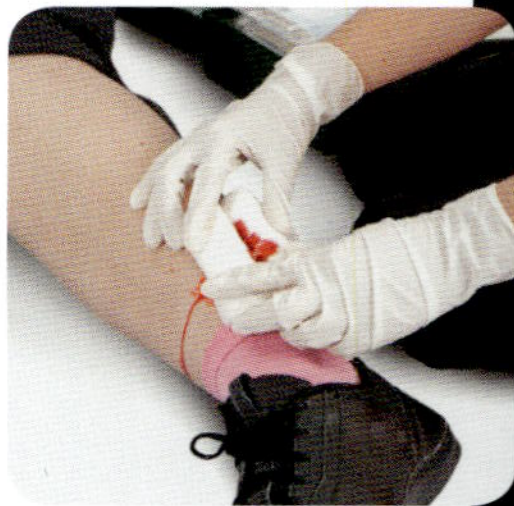

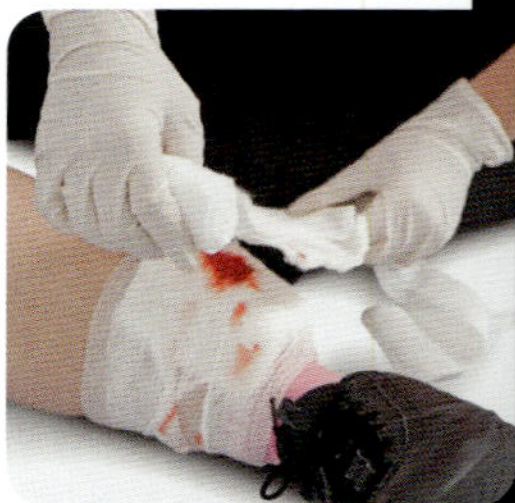

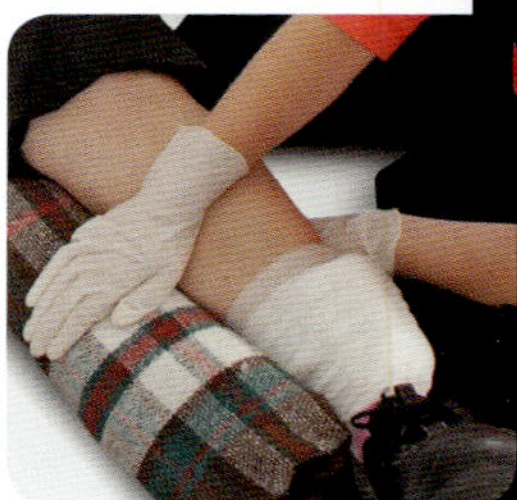

Use broad-fold bandages and ensure that any knots are tied to the uninjured side. Do not wrap a bandage over the fracture. If their circulation is impaired, loosen the dressings

- You MUST NOT try to realign the fracture. This should only be performed by medically trained professionals
- Treat for shock
- Monitor their vital signs
- Do not offer the casualty anything to eat, drink or smoke as a general anaesthetic may have to be administered when they get to hospital

COMPLICATED FRACTURE

Signs and symptoms

- Pain
- Deformity
- Internal and external bleeding
- Shock

Treatment

- Call for an ambulance immediately
- Apply the same treatment as mentioned before for an open or closed fracture
- Be aware of a possible secondary injury which may not be visible. An example of this could be a fractured rib which may have affected an internal organ
- Monitor them very closely and be prepared to resuscitate them

DISLOCATIONS

Dislocations are extremely painful and are often caused by a violent muscle contraction, a strong force wrenching the bone into an abnormal position, or even as something as simple as turning over in bed can cause it.

The recognition of a dislocation is that of a fracture, with the addition of disfigurement around the joint.

In all cases, the ligaments holding the bones together will be damaged.

Under no circumstances should you try to put the dislocated joint back into place.

You must send your casualty to hospital for treatment.

Signs and symptoms

- **Severe pain**
- **Swelling and bruising around the affected joint**
- **Difficulty in moving the affected area**
- **The affected area may look twisted or shortened**

Treatment

If the casualty does not want the limb strapped or supported with an elevated sling, then allow them to support it themselves, if this is possible, and transport them to hospital.

SPRAINS AND STRAINS

These are most commonly associated with sports injuries, or when a person moves suddenly and exerts a great deal of pressure on the muscles or joints. It's sometimes difficult to distinguish between the type of soft tissue injury and a fracture, because of the pain and swelling. If you are unsure, you should suspect the worse and treat for a fracture.

Sprains and strains are collectively known as soft tissue injuries.

SPRAIN

A sprain occurs when one or more of the ligaments have been stretched, twisted, or torn, usually as a result of excessive force being applied to a joint. The most common locations for a sprain to occur are:

- **The knee -** which can become strained when a person turns quickly during sports or other physical activities
- **The ankle -** which can become strained when walking or running on an uneven surface
- **The wrist -** which can become strained when a person falls onto their hand
- **The thumb -** which can become strained during intense and repetitive physical activity, such as playing a racquet sport

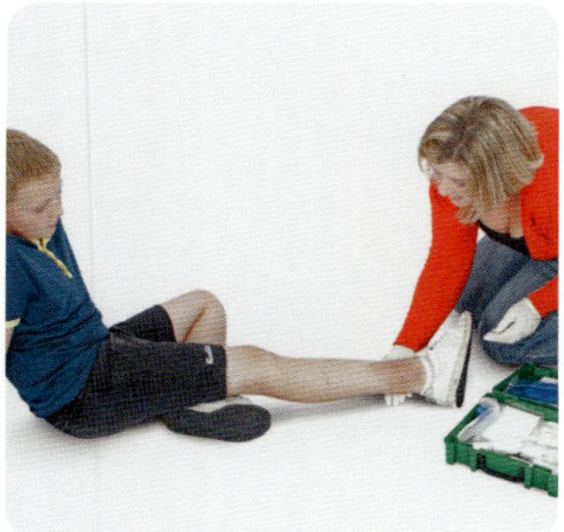

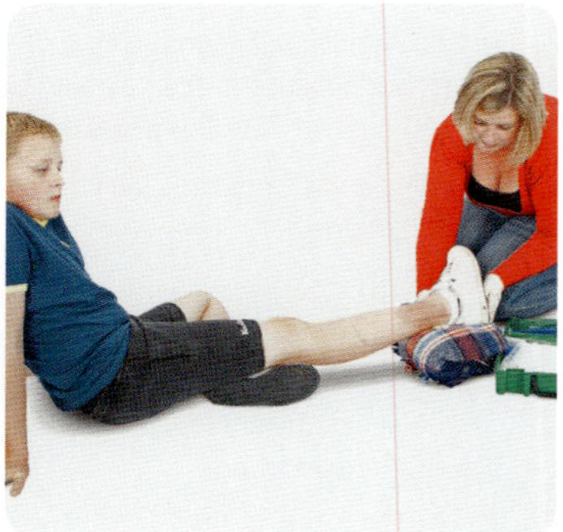

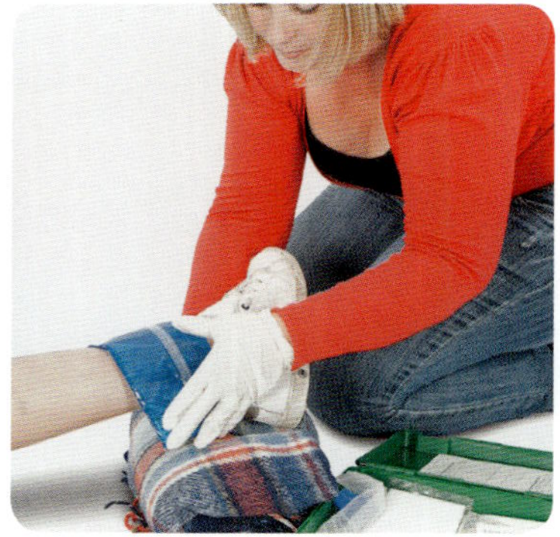

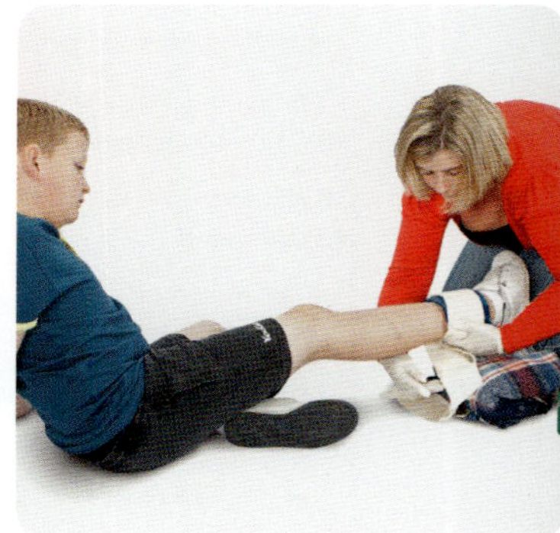

STRAIN

A strain occurs when the muscle fibres stretch or tear. They usually occur for one of two reasons:

- **When the muscle has been stretched beyond its limits**
- **When the muscle has been forced to contract** (shorten too quickly)

Strains can develop as the result of an accident, or during physical or sporting activities, such as running or playing football.

The most common types of strains are:

- **Hamstring strains -** the hamstrings are muscles that run down the back of the leg and are connected to the hip and knee joints
- **Calf muscle strains -** the gastrocnemius and soleus are the medical names for the muscles of the calf located between the ankle and the knee at the back of the leg
- **Quadriceps strains -** the quadriceps are muscles located at the front of the thigh
- **Lumbar strains -** the lumbar muscles are found in the lower back

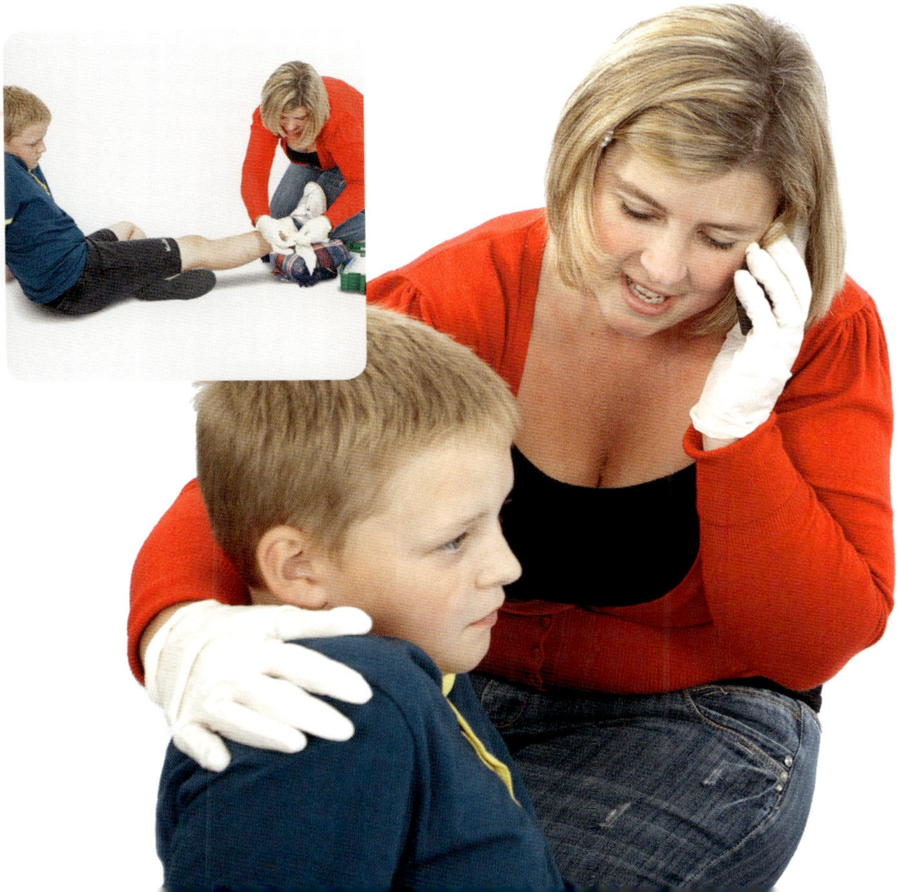

Signs and symptoms for both sprains and strains

- **Pain**
- **Swelling**
- **Bruising**
- **Inflammation**
- **Cramp** (Strains)

Treatment

Firstly, protect the injury from worsening. Asking the casualty to walk or run off the injury could seriously jeopardise the extent of the injury!

PROTECT the injured area from further injury by using a support or (in the case of an ankle injury) wearing shoes that enclose and support the feet, such as lace-ups.

REST by stopping the activity that caused the injury and rest the injured joint or muscle. Avoid activity for the first 48 to 72 hours after the injury was afflicted.

ICE - for the first 48 to 72 hours after the injury, apply ice wrapped in a damp towel to the injured area for 15 to 20 minutes every two to three hours during the day. Do not leave the ice on whilst sleeping, and do not allow the ice to touch the skin directly, because it could cause a cold burn.

COMPRESS or bandage the injured area to limit any swelling and movement that could damage it further. Use a simple elastic bandage or elasticated tubular bandage. It should be wrapped snuggly around the affected area, but not so tightly that it restricts blood flow. Remove the bandage before going to sleep.

ELEVATION - keep the injured area raised and supported to help reduce swelling.

SUPPORT SLING

Fractures to the lower arm and wrist are a common injury. In adults, it accounts for approximately half of all broken bones. In children, fractures of the forearm are second only to broken collarbones.

There is little a First Aider can do other than support it and to dispatch them to hospital.

In respect of support, generally speaking the casualty will support it themselves, and will not want you to move it.

If they are unable to support it themselves, then you can offer to apply a support sling using a triangular bandage.

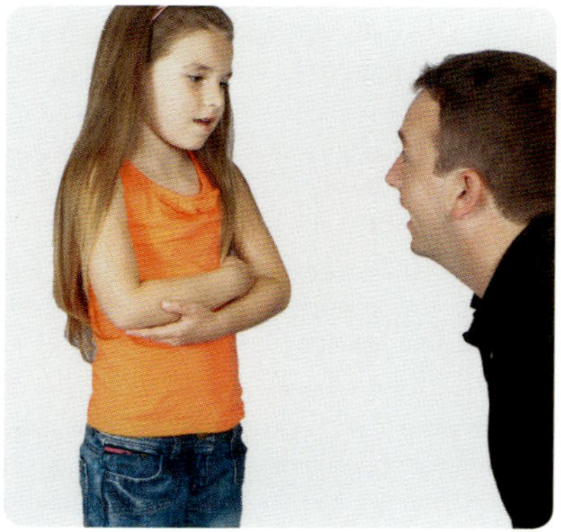

Identify the injury to the arm and providing the arm can be bent at the elbow, offer your casualty a support for it.

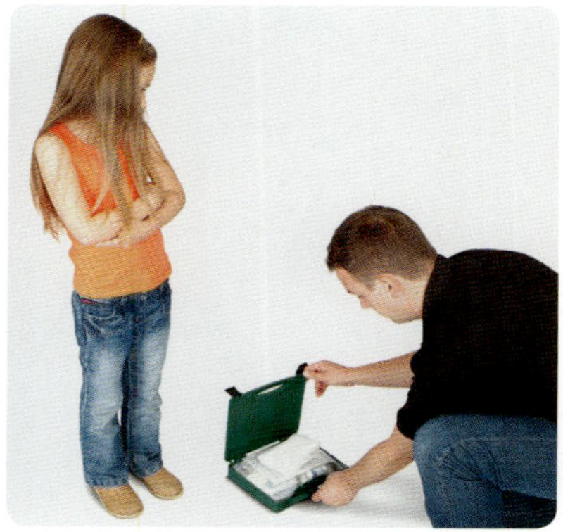

Use a triangular bandage as the support.

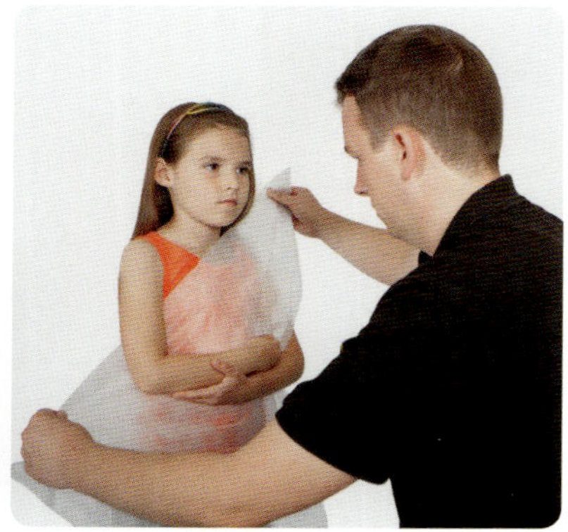

Pass the bandage under the injured arm with the long base running parallel with the body. The point opposite the long base should be at the elbow of the injured arm.

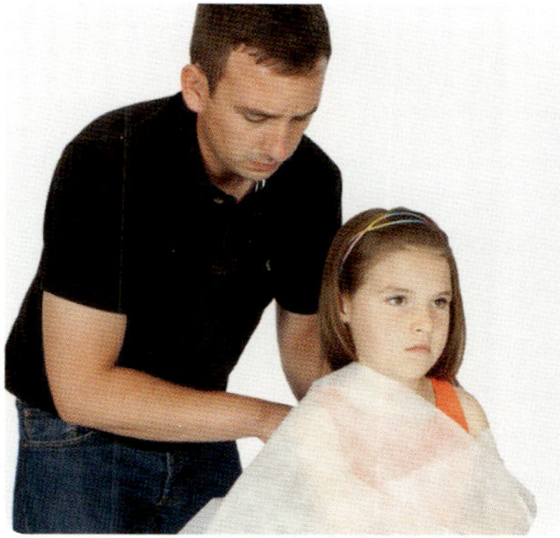

Bring the lower point of the bandage up over the injured arm and over the shoulder so that the two ends meet. Tie off the two ends on the injured side above the collar bone. Place the two ends under the knot to act as a cushion for the knot.

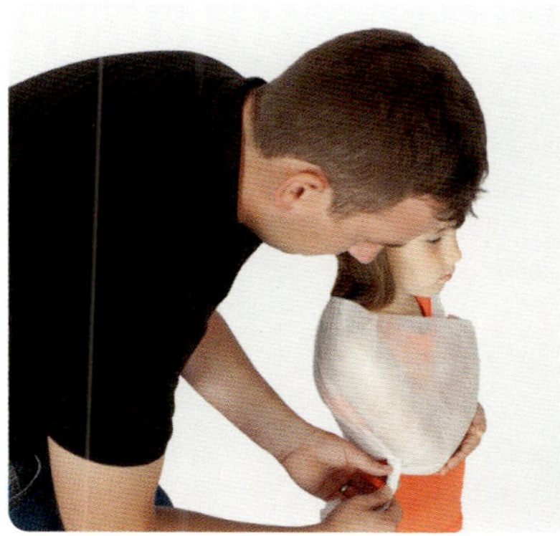

Secure the trailing bandage at the elbow with a safety pin, or by twisting it fairly tight and losing it by tucking it away within the sling.

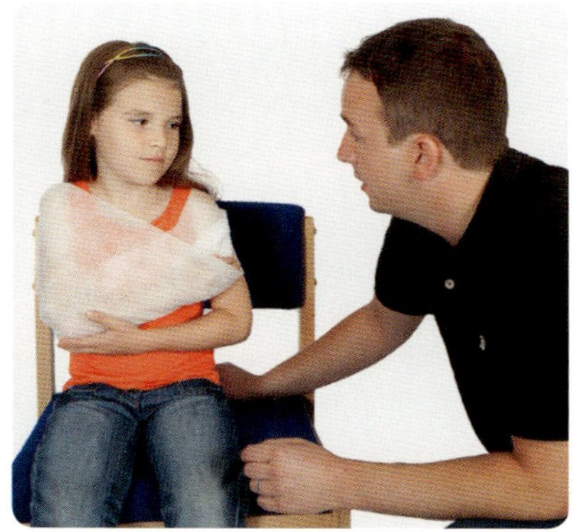

Ensure that there is still circulation in the fingertips by performing a capillary refill check. Press a fingernail which should go pale. When released it should go back to normal colouration. Transport them to the hospital or call 999 if they are unable to walk.

ELEVATED SLING FOR FOREARM AND HAND INJURIES

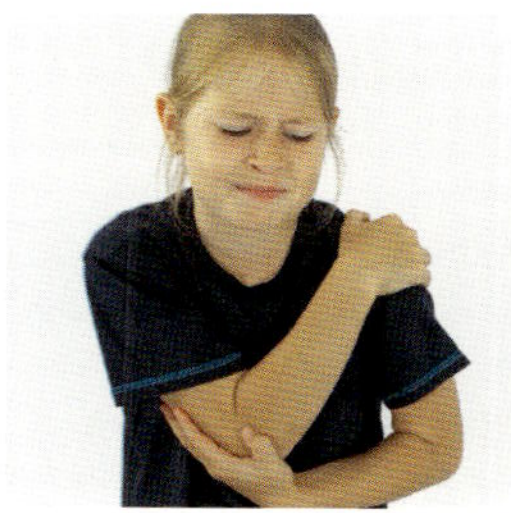

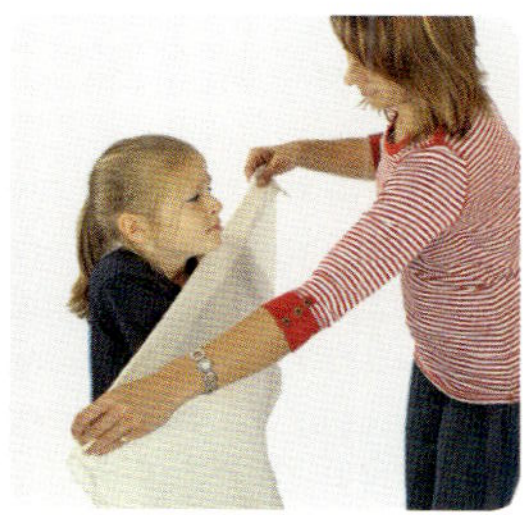

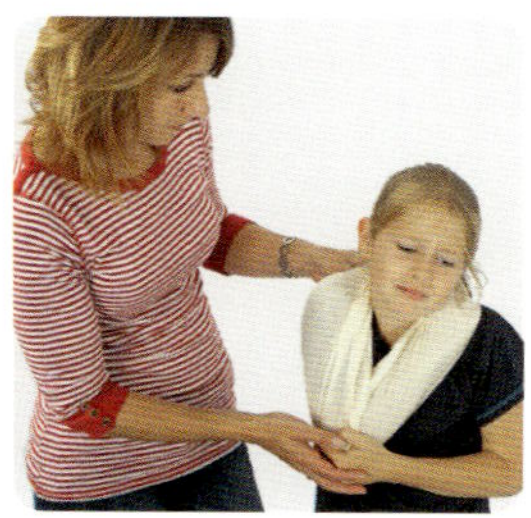

HEAD AND SPINAL INJURIES

If someone is unable to respond to people or activities, then they are deemed as being unresponsive.

Unresponsiveness can be caused by any major illness or injury as well as substance abuse and alcohol use. These conditions include head injuries, poisoning, hypothermia, heatstroke, epilepsy, diabetes, heart attack, stroke and shock. This is by no means the definitive list and this section addresses just some of these conditions.

All injuries to the head are potentially dangerous and they all require a medical assessment.

During any assessment of a head injury, or unresponsiveness, it is useful to record and monitor the casualty by using an observation chart (see page 50).

You should be monitoring and looking at the following:

- **Eyes**
- **Speech**
- **Movement**
- **Breathing**
- **Responsiveness**

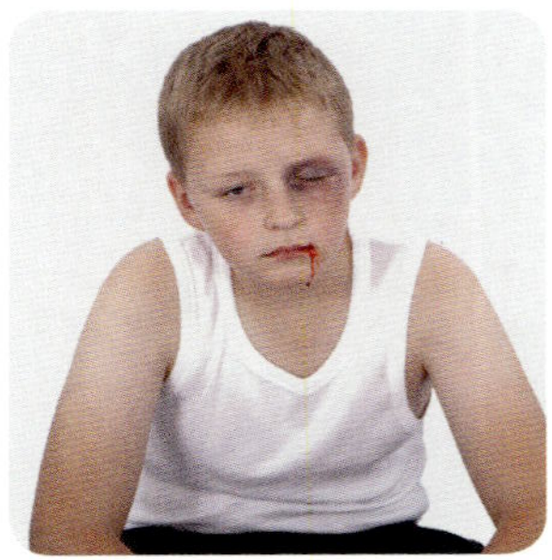

Your objective throughout this monitoring process, is to note any changes in the condition of your casualty in respect of improvement or deterioration.

Although this scale is designed for checks to be made every ten minutes, you should carry out constant monitoring of a casualty until the emergency services take over from you.

CONCUSSION

A concussion is a traumatic brain injury that may result in a bad headache, altered levels of alertness, or unresponsiveness.

It temporarily interferes with the way your brain works, and it can affect memory, judgment, reflexes, speech, balance, coordination, and sleep patterns.

Signs and symptoms

The most common signs and symptoms of concussion are:

- **Evidence of a head injury** (blood or bruising)
- **Headache and nausea**
- **Dizziness and loss of balance**
- **Confusion, such as being unaware of your surroundings**
- **Feeling stunned or dazed**
- **Disturbances with vision, such as double vision or seeing "stars" or flashing lights**
- **Difficulties with memory**

Treatment

- **If they are responsive, rest them by sitting them down, or lying them down with their head raised and hold a cold compress against the injury**
- **Keep them warm and keep talking to them**
- **If they are unresponsive and breathing normally, place them in the recovery position**
- **Monitor their airway, breathing and response levels**
- **If they are unresponsive for more than 3 minutes, you must call for an ambulance**
- **You must recommend that they seek medical advice, particularly if they develop a headache, feel sick or they sleep more than would normally do**

OBSERVATION CHART

The information from this chart will be very valuable when decisions are taken about further treatment

- **Tick the appropriate boxes and update them at ten-minute intervals**
- **Send the completed chart and any notes with the casualty when he or she leaves your care**

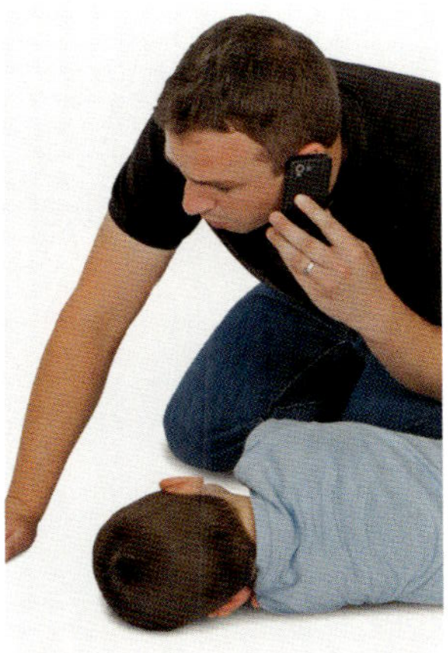

DATE ...... / ...... / ...... CASUALTY'S NAME ....

Time of observation (10-minute intervals)			0	10	20	30	40	50
EYES Observe for reaction while testing other responses	Open spontaneously	4						
	Open to speech	3						
	Open to painful stimulus	2						
	No response	1						
MOVEMENT Apply painful stimulus: pinch the ear lobe or skin on back of hand	Obeys commands	6						
	Points to pain	5						
	Response to painful stimulus	4						
	Bends in response to pain	3						
	Stretches in response to pain	2						
	No response	1						
SPEECH When testing responses, speak clearly and directly, close to casualty's ear	Responds sensibly to questions	5						
	Seems confused	4						
	Uses inappropriate words	3						
	Incomprehensible sounds	2						
	No response	1						
	TOTAL SCORE							
PULSE (Beats per minute) Take pulse at wrist or neck on adult; inner arm on baby	Over 110							
	101-110							
	91-100							
	81-90							
	71-80							
	61-70							
	Below 61							
BREATHING (breaths per minute)	Over 40							
	31-40							
	21-30							
	11-20							
	Below 11							

Note the rate / beats	
Weak = W	
Regular = R	
Strong = S	

Note rate / quality:	
Quiet = Q	
Noisy = N	
Difficult = DIFF	
Easy = E	

SKULL FRACTURE

A skull fracture can be caused by a heavy blow to the head, which may result in a depressed fracture of the skull, or by landing awkwardly from a fall or collision resulting in a base skull fracture. There may also be a wound allowing infection inside the skull. There may also be evidence of concussion and compression.

Signs and symptoms

- **Evidence of trauma to the head**
- **Possible depression of the skull**
- **Bruising around the head**
- **Clear fluid or watery blood coming from the nose or ear**
- **Bloodshot eyes**
- **Deterioration of response levels**

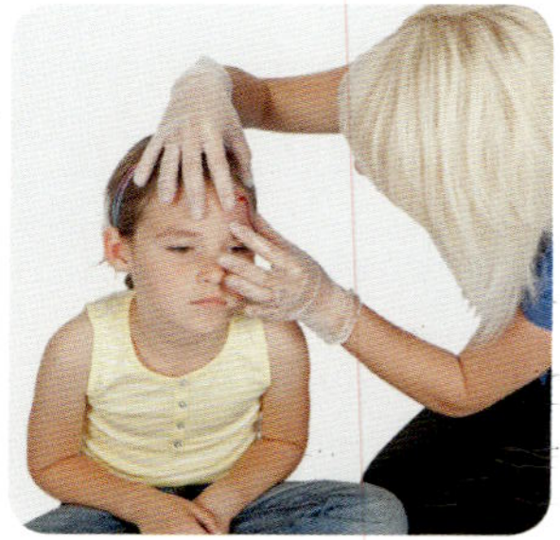

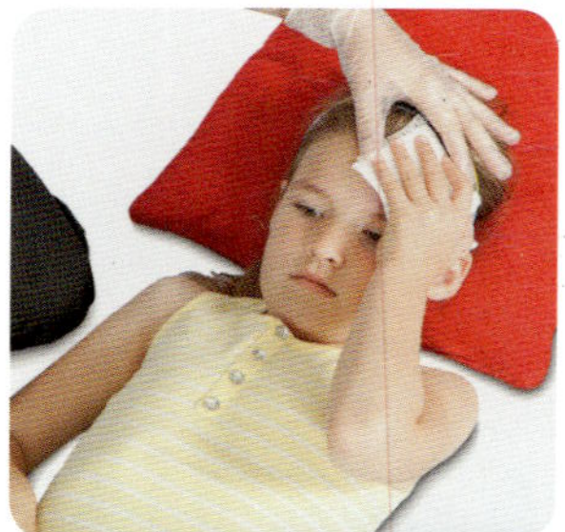

Treatment

- **If you suspect a spinal injury, do not move them**
- **Lay them down, head and shoulders raised if you are able to move them, injured side down**
- **Call for an ambulance**
- **Monitor their airway, breathing and response levels**
- **Cover their ear with a sterile dressing if there is fluid running out of it**
- **Control the bleeding and fluid loss**
- **All head injuries must be advised to go to hospital**

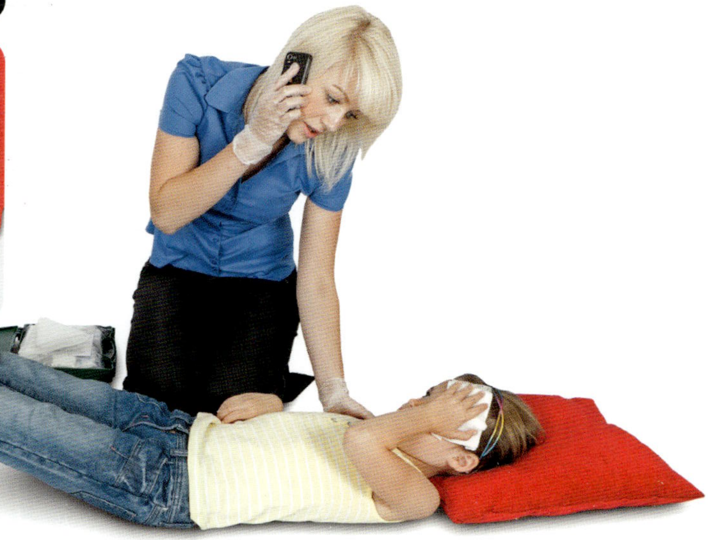

CEREBRAL COMPRESSION

This very serious condition is due to pressure being exerted on the brain from a build-up of blood or fluid, blood clot, or depressed as a result of a skull fracture.

This may follow on from concussion either directly, or at some point after their apparent recovery. For this reason, all head injuries must be examined by medical personnel.

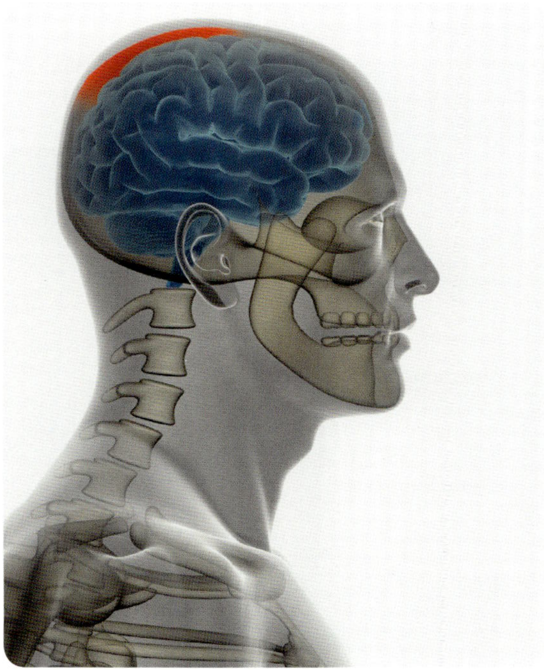

Signs and symptoms

- Their response levels will deteriorate, possibly leading to unresponsiveness
- Signs of a recent head injury
- Severe headache
- Weakness and/or paralysis down one side of the face or body
- Flushed face and high temperature
- Drowsiness
- Behavioural changes
- Slow noisy breathing
- Unequal pupil sizes

Treatment

- Call for an ambulance immediately
- If they are responsive, keep them supported in a comfortable position by lying them down with their head and shoulders raised, providing injuries allow, and keeping them warm
- Monitor their response levels
- If they become unresponsive, check their breathing and carry out your basic life support procedures dependant on the result

SPINAL INJURIES

The spine, also known as the backbone, is a strong, flexible column of ring-like bones that runs from our skull to our pelvis. It holds the head and body upright and allows us to bend and twist our body. It also offers protection to our spinal cord - a large bundle of nerves that runs through the cavity in the centre of our spine that relays messages between our brain and the rest of our body.

It is made up of 33 irregularly shaped bones called vertebrae.

Each vertebra has a hole in the middle through which the spinal cord runs.

The spine can be divided into five different regions, from top to bottom:

1. **Seven cervical vertebrae support our head and neck and allow us to nod and shake our head**
2. **Our ribs are attached to our 12 thoracic vertebrae**
3. **Our five sturdy lumbar vertebrae carry most of the weight of our upper body and provide a stable centre of gravity when we move**
4. **Our sacrum is made up of five fused vertebrae. It makes up the back wall of our pelvis**
5. **Our coccyx is made up of four fused vertebrae. It is an evolutionary remnant of the tail found in most other vertebrates**

Shock absorbers

Sandwiched between our vertebrae are pads of tough, fibrous cartilage called inter-vertebral discs that cushion our vertebrae and absorb shock. These discs, together with the curved 'S' shape of our spine, prevents shock to our head when we walk or run.

Any damage to our spine can not only be life-threatening, but it can also leave us permanently damaged. It can lead to paralysis to parts of our body that is irreparable.

Therefore, your handling of your casualty where you suspect a spinal injury is critical in ensuring that their condition does not worsen.

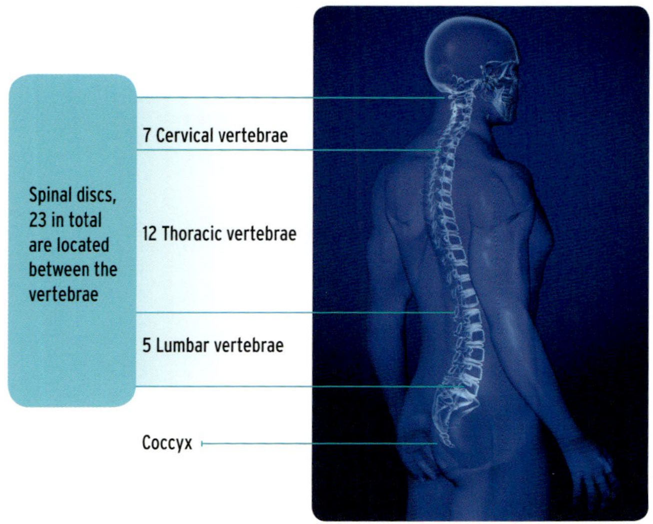

Signs and symptoms

When the spinal column or vertebrae are damaged:

- **An unusual curvature of the spine**
- **Pain at the site of injury. Be aware that this may be masked by other pains in other parts of the body**
- **Tenderness in the skin that covers the spine**

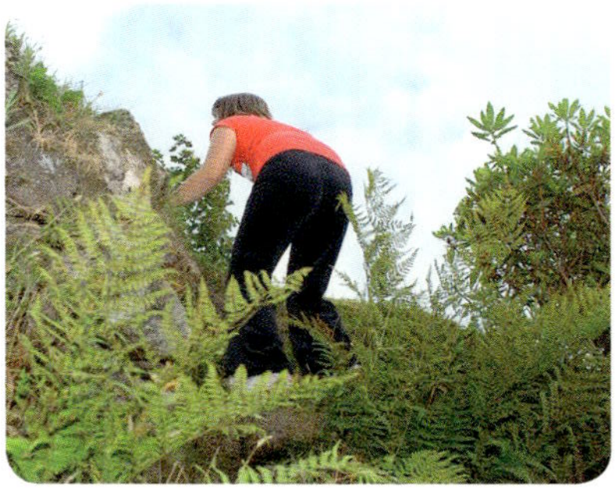

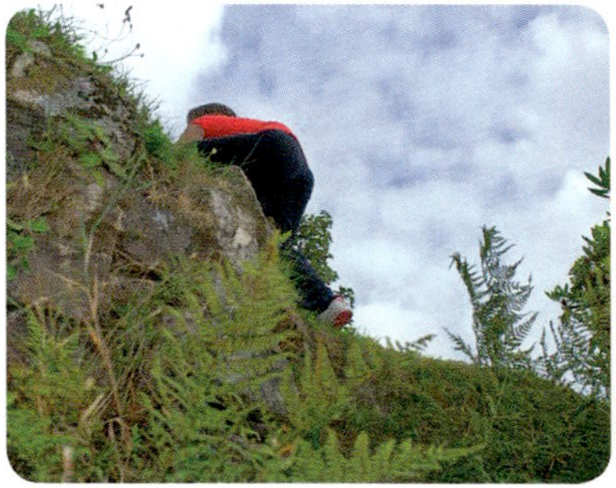

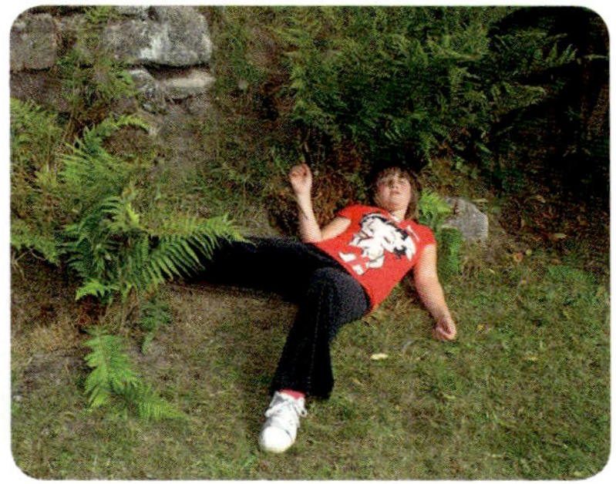

When the spinal cord is damaged:

- **No control over limb movement**
- **Loss of sensation, or abnormal sensations such as numbness, burning or tingling**
- **The casualty may say that the limbs feel heavy or clumsy**
- **Loss of bladder and bowel control**
- **Breathing difficulties**

Treatment

- **Call for an ambulance immediately**
- **Prevent any movement and support in the position found**
- **Monitor their breathing and be prepared to resuscitate**

FOREIGN BODY AND EYE INJURIES

THE NOSE

- **Objects pushed up the nose may cause blockages or infection**
  Keep your casualty calm and reassure them.
- **Get the casualty to breathe through their mouth**
- **Do not attempt to remove the object**
- **Send the casualty to hospital**

THE EARS

If a foreign object enters the ear and becomes lodged, it can cause damage to the ear canal, the eardrum and in some cases, cause temporary deafness.

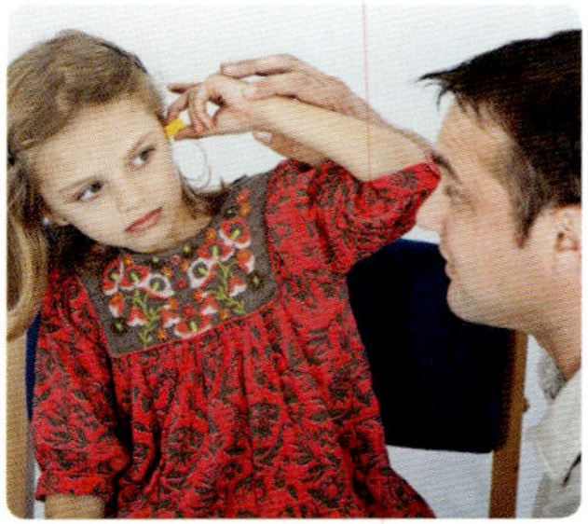

The object should be left in the ear, unless it's a living object such as an insect that could be removed by flooding the ear with tepid water.

If this doesn't work, then you must seek medical advice.

If you need to seek medical advice:

- **Cover the ear with a sterile dressing, taking care not to put any direct pressure on the object**
- **Send the casualty to hospital**

SWALLOWED OBJECTS

Small objects are commonly swallowed by children. Many will enter the digestive system without choking the casualty, and leave the body in its natural way. However, you should seek medical attention irrespective. If you know that the object was sharp or toxic, then you must seek urgent medical attention.

If the object becomes stuck in the respiratory tract, then you should follow the choking procedure.

Some sharp objects may stick in the throat, such as fish bones or glass. If this is the case, then you must seek urgent medical attention as the airway could swell which would affect the casualty's ability to breathe normally.

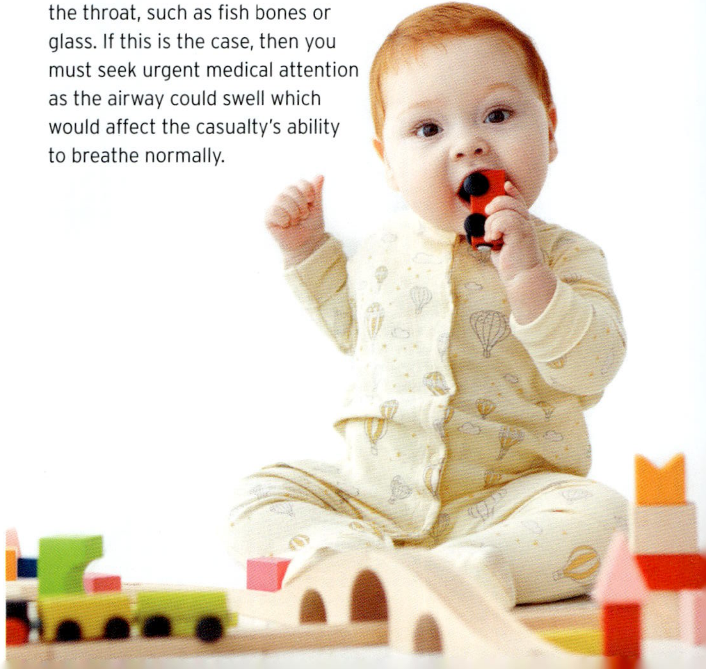

EYE INJURIES

Eye injuries have a number of different causes, such as a blow to the eye, foreign bodies, lacerations (cuts) and ultraviolet light.

Eye injuries can also be caused by chemical exposures and burns as a result of liquid being splashed into the eyes.

Some aerosols can be harmful to the eyes, including Mace (attack defence spray), tear gas, pepper spray and some chemicals in hair spray. Chemicals can also be transferred from the skin on your hands to your eyes.

A BLOW TO THE EYE

Serious and permanent eye damage can result from a blunt object, from a sports injury, a fall or a fight. Care should be taken when treating such an injury as the bone surrounding the eye could be fractured.

Signs and symptoms

- **Pain**
- **Swelling**
- **Bruising**
- **Possible bleeding**
- **Redness of the eye**
- **Headache**

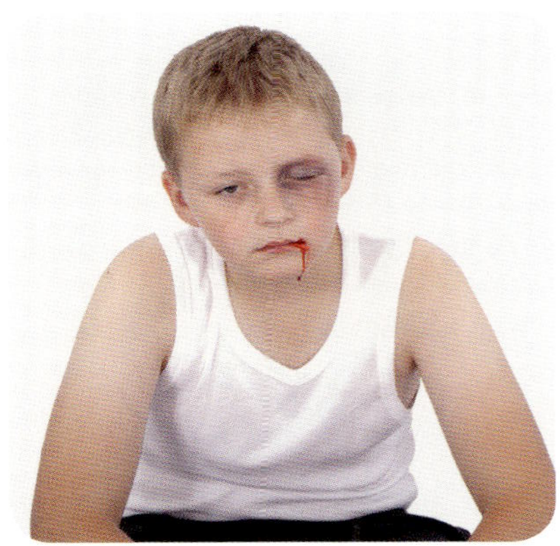

Treatment

When to seek medical help.

Send your casualty to see their GP if:

- **They have a change in vision**
- **The pain is persistent**
- **There is pus or warmth and redness, indicating infection**
- **They become forgetful or drowsy**
- **They have nausea, vomiting and/or dizziness**
- **The swelling does not subside after a few days**

Go to your hospital accident and emergency department if:

- **They have two black eyes (this could suggest a skull fracture)**
- **They have double vision**
- **They cannot move the eye**
- **They think something has pierced the eye**
- **There is a cut to the eye or blood inside the eye**
- **Fluid is leaking from the eye or the eye looks deformed**
- **They are taking blood-thinning medication such as aspirin, or have a bleeding disorder such as haemophilia**

FOREIGN BODY AND EYE INJURIES continued

FOREIGN BODIES IN THE EYE

Foreign bodies, such as metal, plastic or wood, can scratch or graze the surface of the eye or cornea.

Examples of foreign bodies that can cause a corneal abrasion include being poked in the eye by a finger or hot cigarette ash flying into the eye.

In severe cases, the foreign body may be embedded.

Signs and symptoms

- **Sensation that something is in the eye**
- **Increase in tears produced by the eye**
- **Pain**
- **Blurred or double vision**
- **Sensitivity to light**
- **A visible foreign body on the cornea**
- **A rust ring or stain on the cornea if the foreign body is metal**

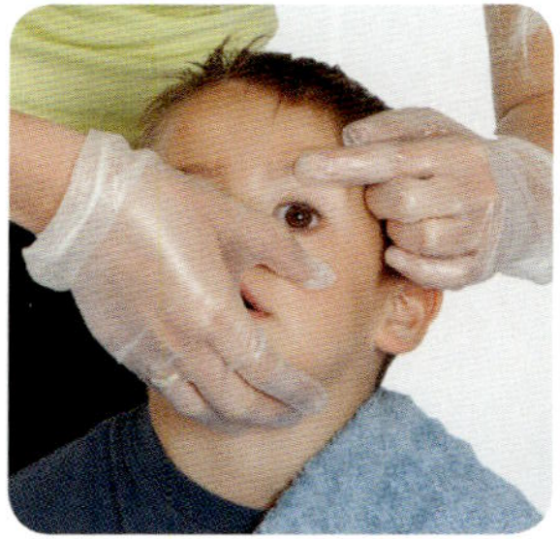

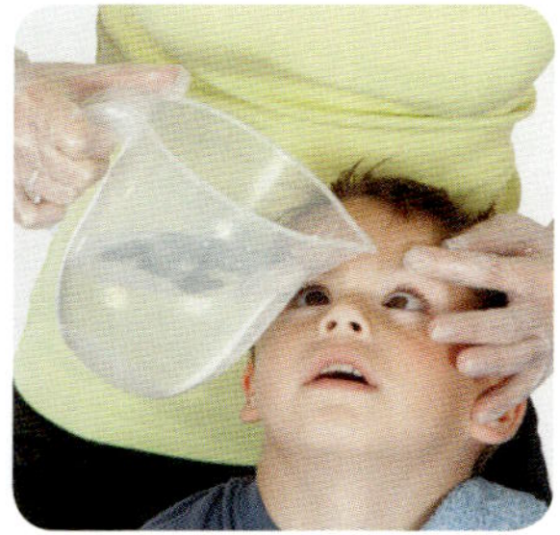

Treatment

- **Sit the casualty down, and stand behind them**
- **Lean their head back and very gently separate their eyelid with your finger and thumb and inspect the eye**

If there is something embedded, then you must leave it in place. Cover the eye with a sterile dressing, being extremely careful not to make any contact with the foreign body that is embedded. Transport them to hospital immediately, or ring for an ambulance.

- **If you can see the foreign object, then try flushing it out with a sterile eye wash solution, or clean tap water. Place a towel on the shoulder on the side of the injured eye. Lean the head back and inclined towards the injured side. Gently pour the eye wash into the eye to flush it out**
- **If this hasn't worked, then use the corner of a tissue or handkerchief, moisten it and try to remove it by using the point**
- **If this doesn't work, then you must seek medical advice**

LACERATIONS

Eye lacerations can be caused by falls, contact with sharp objects, particularly flying objects such as grit, debris from a garden strimmer and shards of glass.

Signs and symptoms

- **Eye pain and sensitivity to light**
- **Increase in tears produced by the eye**
- **Blurred or distorted vision**
- **Squinting caused by spasm of the muscle surrounding the eye**
- **Feeling that something is in the eye and it cannot be removed**

Treatment

- **Lie the casualty down and support their head in order to rest them. Try to keep both their eyes still**
- **Cover their injured eye with a sterile eye dressing, or ask them to hold a sterile dressing in place**
- **Take them to the hospital if you are able to transport them. Failing that, call for an ambulance immediately**

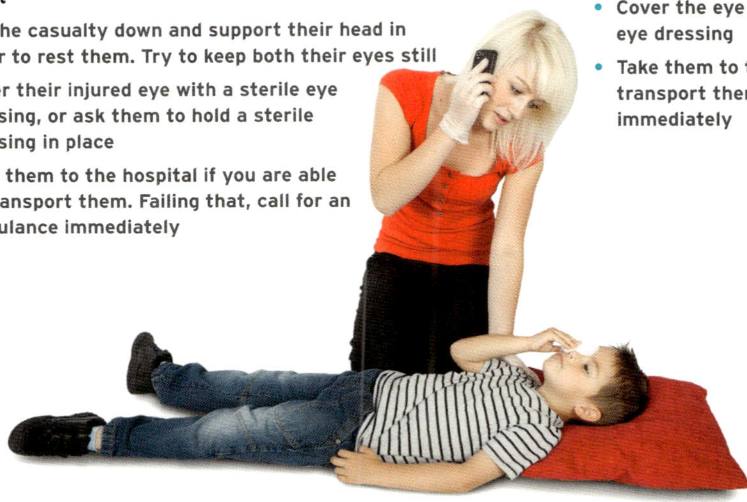

ULTRAVIOLET LIGHT

Ultraviolet (UV) light can lead to an eye injury called corneal flash burn.

Exposure to the sun, glare from a welder's torch and sun lamps can cause of this type of injury. It could also affect both eyes.

Signs and symptoms

- **Pain**
- **Redness and watering**
- **A gritty feeling**
- **Sensitive to light**

Treatment

- **Cover the eye with a sterile eye dressing**
- **Take them to the hospital if you are able to transport them. Failing that, call for an ambulance immediately**

CHEMICAL BURNS

The surface of the eye can be severely damaged with any type of chemical burn. It can lead to the loss of sight if it is not treated quickly.

Chemicals can be transferred to the eye by splashing, spraying or simply from your own finger should it be contaminated.

Signs and symptoms

- **Watering of the eye**
- **Pain**
- **Swelling**
- **Redness**
- **Evidence of the chemical**

Treatment

- **You must wear gloves to prevent yourself being contaminated by the chemical**
- **Irrigate the eye for 10 minutes under running cool water, either by holding the head under a running tap, or by flushing the eye with a continual supply of cool tap water from a suitable container**
- **Ensure that the irrigation does not flow into the other eye**
- **Try to identify the chemical so that the emergency services know what chemical they are treating**
- **Cover the injured eye with a sterile eye dressing**
- **Arrange to transport them to hospital, or call for an ambulance**

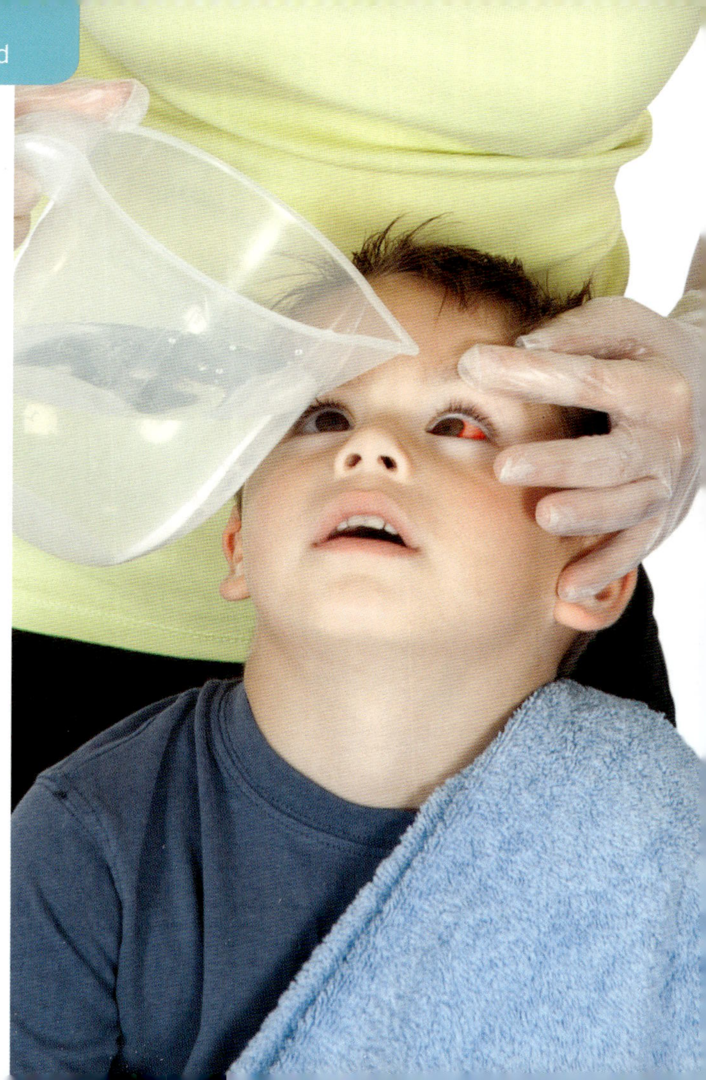

SICKLE CELL ANAEMIA

Sickle cell anaemia is a genetic (inherited) blood disorder where red blood cells develop abnormally.

Red blood cells carry oxygen from the lungs to the rest of the body. The cells are usually round and flexible, allowing them to move easily around the body.

However, in people with sickle cell anaemia, the shape and texture of the blood cells can change. They become hard and sticky and are shaped like sickles (crescents). The cells die prematurely, leading to a shortage of red blood cells. This causes symptoms of anaemia, such as tiredness and breathlessness. The sticky red blood cells can clog up blood vessels, resulting in nearby tissue becoming starved of oxygen. The lack of oxygen can trigger episodes of moderate to severe pain. These episodes are known as a sickle cell crisis.

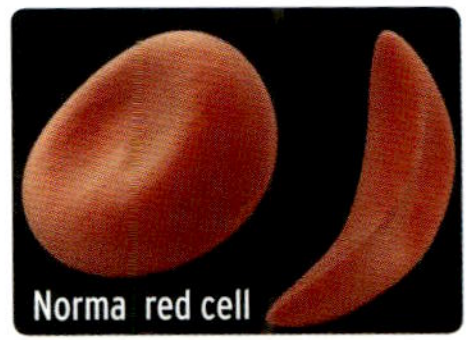

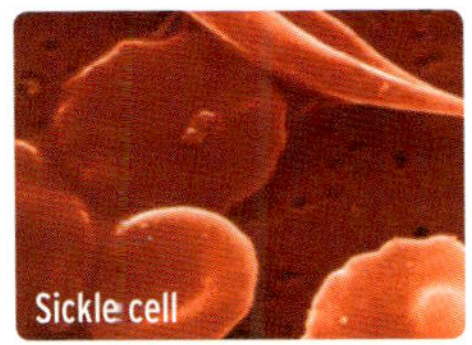

A lack of a regular oxygen supply can also result in tissue and organ damage.

This can potentially lead to a wide range of complications, including:

- **A stroke, where the blood supply to the brain is interrupted**
- **Frequent and often serious infections because the spleen, which plays an important part in fighting infection, becomes damaged**

Acute chest syndrome, a serious and sometimes life-threatening lung condition, which is thought to be triggered by infection.

Signs and symptoms

Sickle cell anaemia can cause a wide range of symptoms. However, not everyone with the condition will experience all the symptoms described below.

- **Fatigue**
- **Shortness of breath**
- **Pain in the chest, bones and tummy**
- **Palpitations (irregular heartbeat)**

Your child's body is usually able to compensate for the lack of red blood cells by an increase in heartbeat, although the symptoms of fatigue and a general lack of stamina may persist.

This can make participating in physical activities, such as sports, more difficult for your child.

Treatment

- **Ensure that they drink plenty of fluids. Fluids can help thin the blood and clear out the sickle cells that are clogging the blood vessels**
- **Place them in a warm bath. Ensure that the water is not too hot and do not let it get too cold because changes in temperature could trigger another crisis**
- **Use suitable distractions. For example, reading them a story, watching a DVD or playing their favourite computer game will help to take their mind of the pain**
- **Summon an ambulance if the pain becomes too great**

DIABETES

Diabetes is a long-term condition caused by too much glucose, a type of sugar, in the blood. It is also known as diabetes mellitus.

Normally, the amount of sugar in the blood is controlled by a hormone called insulin. Insulin is produced by the pancreas, a gland located behind the stomach. When food is digested and enters the bloodstream, insulin helps move any glucose out of the blood and into cells, where it is broken down to produce energy.

For people with diabetes, the body is unable to break down glucose into energy. This is because there is either not enough insulin to move the glucose, or because the insulin that is there does not work properly.

There are two types of diabetes:

Type 1 diabetes occurs when the body produces no insulin. It is often referred to as insulin-dependent diabetes, juvenile diabetes or early-onset diabetes because it usually develops before the age of 40, often during the teenage years.

Type 1 diabetes is far less common than type 2 diabetes, and make up only 10% of all people with diabetes who will have to take insulin injections for life.

Type 2 diabetes occurs when not enough insulin is produced by the body for it to function properly, or when the body's cells do not react to insulin. This is called insulin resistance.

General signs and symptoms

- **Feeling very thirsty**
- **Going to the toilet a lot, especially at night**
- **Extreme tiredness**
- **Weight loss and muscle wasting**
  (loss of muscle bulk)

Hyperglycaemia occurs when there is a higher than normal level of glucose (sugar) in the blood.

This causes:

- **Increased thirst**
- **The need to urinate frequently**
- **Tiredness**

Hypoglycaemia means that there is an abnormally low level of sugar (glucose) in the blood.

When the glucose level is too low - called a 'hypo' - the body does not have enough energy to carry out its activities.

Most people will have some warning that their blood glucose levels are too low, which will give them time to correct it.

Typical early warning signs are:

- **Feeling hungry**
- **Trembling or shakiness**
- **Sweating**

Treatment

Hyperglycaemia

Hyperglycaemia is the medical term for a high blood sugar (glucose) level.

- **Call for an ambulance**
- **If they become unresponsive, place them in the recovery position**
- **Monitor their breathing and response levels**

Signs & Symptoms	HYPERglycaemia	HYPOglycaemia
Amount of insulin used	Not enough	Too much
Deterioration	Gradual	Very quick
Hunger	Absent	Present
Vomiting	Common	Uncommon
Thirst	Present	Absent
Breath odour	Fruity/sweet	Normal
Pulse	Rapid and weak	Rapid and strong
Breathing	Rapid	Normal
Skin	Dry and warm	Pale, cold and sweaty
Seizures	Uncommon	Common
Responsiveness	Drowsy	Rapid loss

Treatment

Hypoglycaemia

A low blood sugar, or a "hypo", is where the level of sugar (glucose) in your blood drops too low.

- **Sit the casualty down**
- **Offer them 15-20gms of glucose.**
  Offer a sugary drink or sweet food if glucose is not available
- **Monitor and reassure them**
- **Call for an ambulance if the above is ineffective**
- **If they become unresponsive, place them in the recovery position and monitor them**

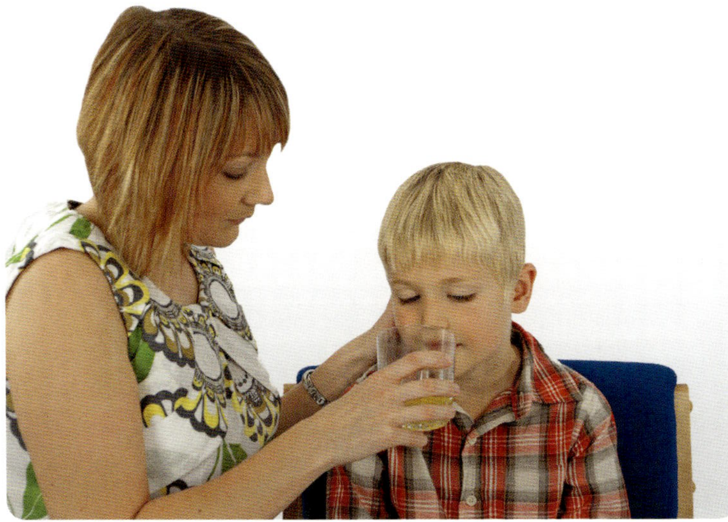

ASTHMA

Asthma is a common long-term condition that can be well controlled in most children.

The severity of asthma symptoms varies between children, from very mild to more severe.

In the UK, over 1.1 million children have asthma. It is more common in young boys than young girls. However, this changes as children get older and, after puberty, asthma is more common in girls.

During the teenage years, the symptoms of asthma may disappear. However, asthma can return in adulthood. If the childhood symptoms of asthma are moderate to severe, it is less likely that the condition will get better in adolescence and more likely that it will return later in life.

The cause of asthma is not fully understood. It is known that asthma often runs in families and a child is more likely to have asthma if one or both parents have the condition.

What is asthma?

Asthma affects the airways, the small tubes that carry air in and out of the lungs (known as the bronchi). If your child has asthma, the airways of their lungs are more sensitive than normal. When your child comes into contact with something that irritates their lungs, known as a trigger, their airways become narrow, the lining becomes inflamed, the muscles around them tighten, and there is an increase in the production of sticky mucus or phlegm. This makes it difficult to breathe and causes wheezing, coughing, shortness of breath and can make the chest feel tight.

A sudden, severe onset of symptoms is known as an asthma attack, or an acute asthma exacerbation. Asthma attacks can sometimes be managed at home but may require hospital treatment. They are occasionally life threatening.

Common triggers

A trigger is anything that irritates the airways and causes the symptoms of asthma. Everyone's asthma is different and people may have several triggers.

The most common trigger of an asthma attack is having an upper respiratory tract infection, such as a cold or flu. Other common triggers include:

- **Exercise, especially in cold weather**
- **An allergy to and contact with house dust mites, animal fur, grass and tree pollen**
- **Exposure to air pollution, especially tobacco smoke**

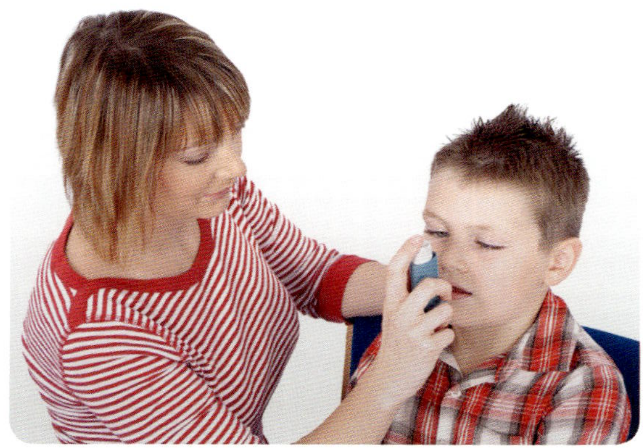

The common symptoms of asthma include:

- **Feeling breathless**
- **Wheezing** (there may be a whistling sound when your child breathes)
- **Coughing, particularly at night**
- **Tightness in the chest**

Symptoms vary between people and children may have one or more of these symptoms. If symptoms become worse during the night or with exercise, your child's asthma may not be well controlled. Take your child to see their doctor or asthma nurse.

Treatment

The aim of the treatment is to get your child's asthma under control and keep it that way.

Asthma treatments are effective in most children and should allow them to be free from symptoms and lead a normal life.

Your doctor or nurse will tailor your child's asthma treatment according to their symptoms. Sometimes, your child may need to be on higher levels of medication than at other times.

You and your child should be offered:

- **Care at your GP surgery from doctors and nurses trained in asthma management**
- **Advice about the risks to you and your children with asthma if you smoke, as well as support to stop smoking**
- **Vaccinations to reduce respiratory infections, such as flu**
- **A written personal asthma action plan agreed with your child's doctor or nurse**

NB: Schools are now allowed to keep an emergency inhaler close to the First Aid kit. It is permissable to offer this treatment in an emergency.

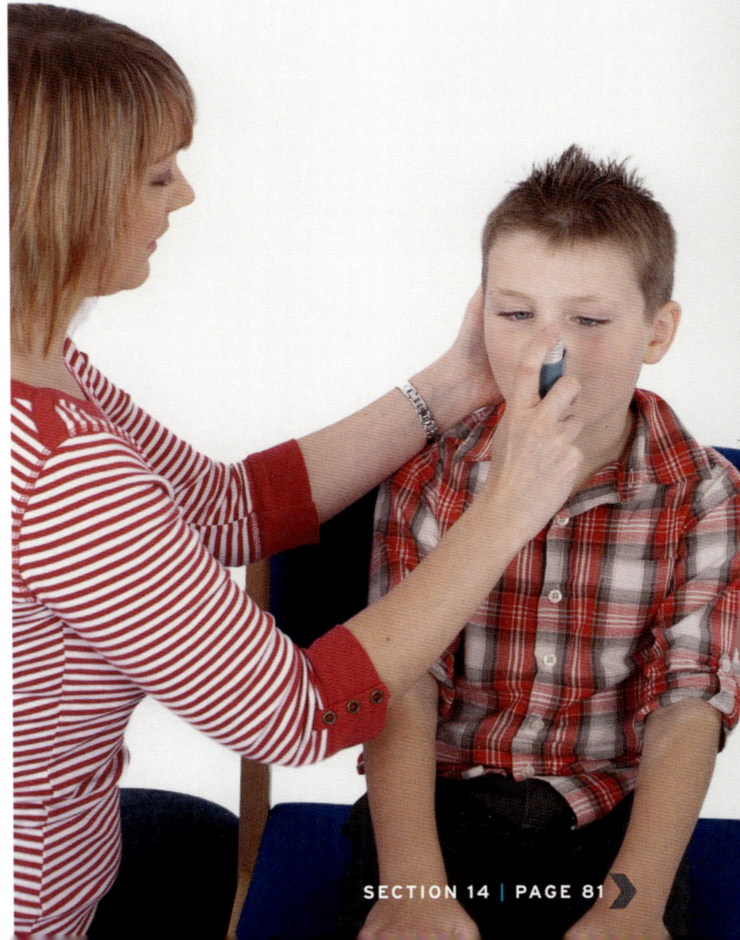

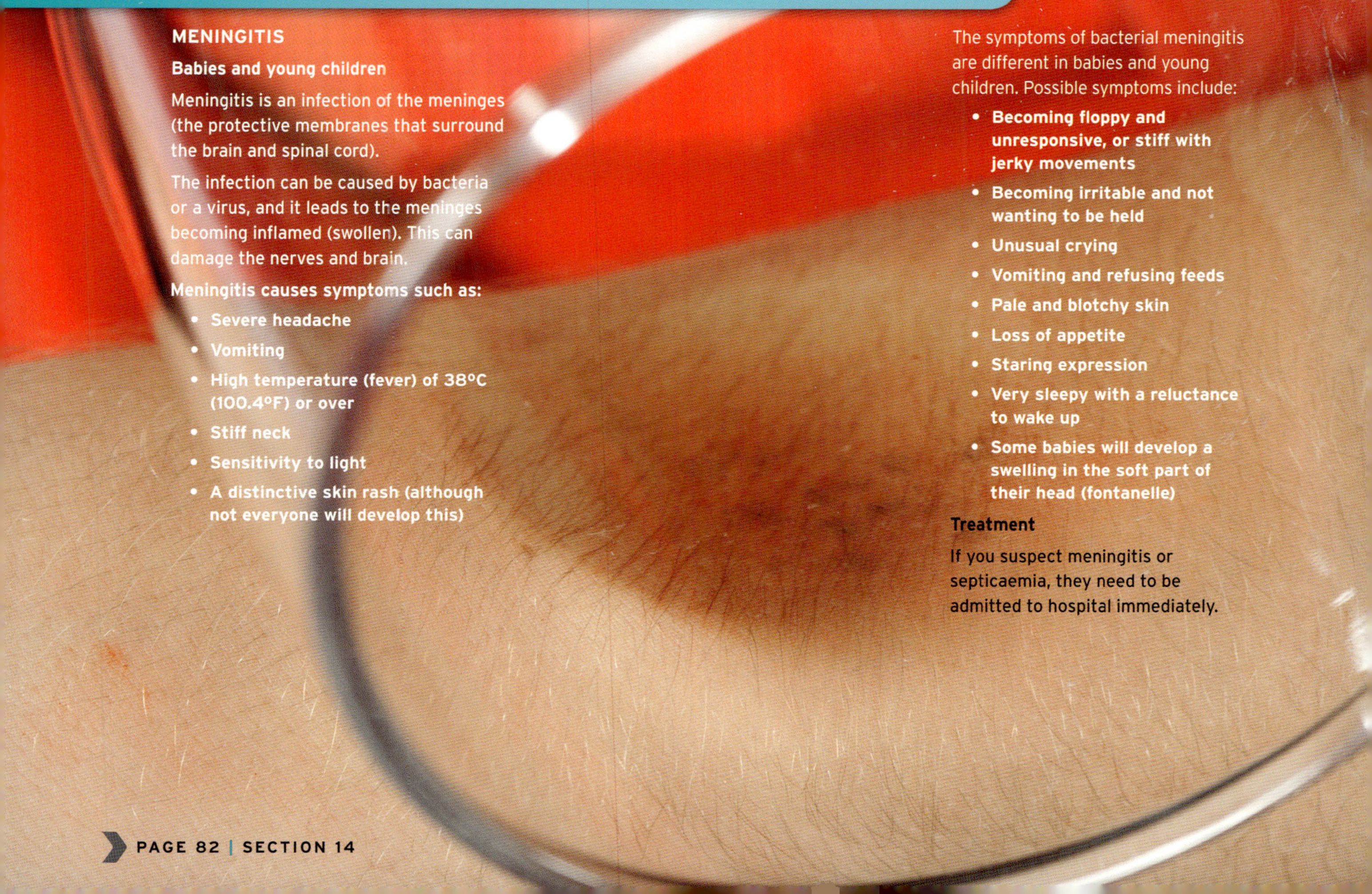

MENINGITIS

Babies and young children

Meningitis is an infection of the meninges (the protective membranes that surround the brain and spinal cord).

The infection can be caused by bacteria or a virus, and it leads to the meninges becoming inflamed (swollen). This can damage the nerves and brain.

Meningitis causes symptoms such as:

- **Severe headache**
- **Vomiting**
- **High temperature (fever) of 38°C (100.4°F) or over**
- **Stiff neck**
- **Sensitivity to light**
- **A distinctive skin rash (although not everyone will develop this)**

The symptoms of bacterial meningitis are different in babies and young children. Possible symptoms include:

- **Becoming floppy and unresponsive, or stiff with jerky movements**
- **Becoming irritable and not wanting to be held**
- **Unusual crying**
- **Vomiting and refusing feeds**
- **Pale and blotchy skin**
- **Loss of appetite**
- **Staring expression**
- **Very sleepy with a reluctance to wake up**
- **Some babies will develop a swelling in the soft part of their head (fontanelle)**

Treatment

If you suspect meningitis or septicaemia, they need to be admitted to hospital immediately.

FEBRILE CONVULSIONS

Febrile convulsions, or seizures, are a relatively common childhood condition, referring to a child having a seizure (fit) when they have a high temperature of 38°C (100.4°F) or above. This is usually the result of an infection.

Witnessing a child having a seizure, particularly if they have no previous history of them, can be very frightening and distressing for you.

Many parents who have witnessed their child having a febrile seizure say they were convinced that their child was going to die. However, although febrile seizures may be very frightening, most are harmless and do not pose a threat to a child's health.

Febrile seizures often occur during the first day of a fever, which is defined as a high temperature of 38°C (100.4°F) or above.

Seizures can develop even after a mild temperature, and may not develop at all with an extremely high temperature.

Simple febrile seizures can sometimes occur at the time of a rapid rise in temperature. In these cases, it is common to only realise that your child is ill when they have the seizure.

Alternatively, seizures can occur as their temperature drops from a previously high level.

During simple febrile seizures, their body will become stiff and their arms and legs will begin to twitch. They will lose responsiveness and they may wet or soil themselves. They may also vomit and foam at the mouth. The seizure usually lasts for less than five minutes.

Following a febrile seizure, they may be sleepy for up to an hour afterwards.

Treatment

- **Place them in the recovery position. This will stop them swallowing any vomit, and it will keep their airway open and help to prevent injury**
- **Stay with them and make a note of when the seizure started in order to keep track of how long it lasts**
- **If the seizure lasts for less than five minutes, phone your GP or NHS Direct on 111**
- **Avoid putting anything in your child's mouth while they are having a seizure**
- **If the seizure lasts for longer than five minutes, dial 999 to ask for an ambulance to take your child to the nearest hospital**

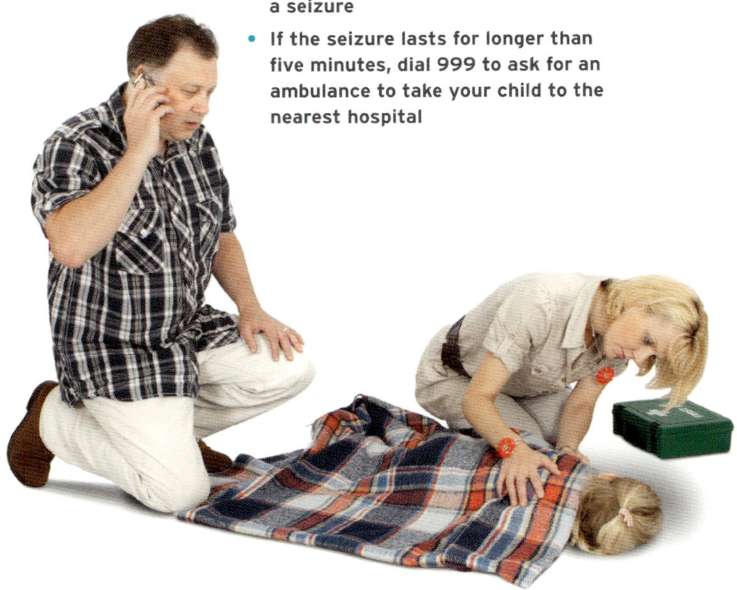

EFFECTS OF EXTREME HEAT AND COLD

HEAT EXHAUSTION

Heat exhaustion is brought on when the temperature inside the body, known as the core temperature, rises from the normal 37°c up to 40°c (98.6-104°F). At that temperature, the levels of water and salt in the body begin to drop. This causes symptoms such as nausea, feeling faint and heavy sweating.

If it is left untreated, heat exhaustion can sometimes lead to heatstroke.

Signs and symptoms

- **The skin will be feeling very hot and flushed**
- **Heavy sweating**
- **Dizziness**
- **Fatigue**
- **Nausea**
- **Vomiting**
- **Rapid heartbeat**
- **Mental confusion**
- **Urinating less often and the colour of the urine being much darker than usual**

Treatment

- **Get them to rest in a cool place,** ideally in a room with air conditioning, or at least somewhere that is in the shade
- **Give them plenty of fluids to drink.** This should either be water or a rehydration drink such as a sports drink. Avoid alcohol or caffeine as this can increase dehydration
- **Cool their skin with cold water.** If available, use a shower or cold bath to cool them down. If not, then apply wet towels to their skin
- **Loosen any unnecessary clothing,** and make sure that the person gets plenty of air

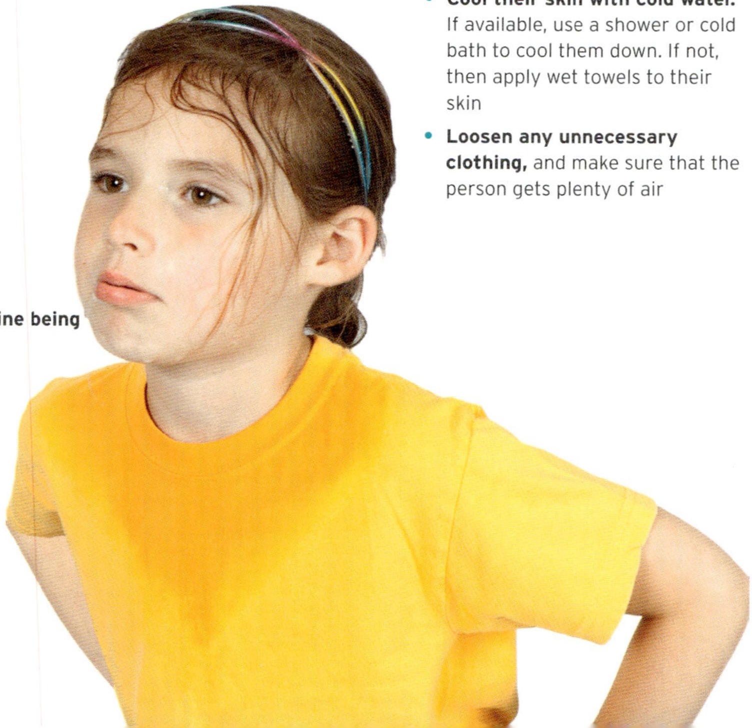

HEATSTROKE

Heatstroke happens when a person's core temperature rises above 40°C (104°F). Cells inside the body begin to break down and important parts of the body stop working.

Symptoms of heatstroke can include mental confusion, hyperventilation (rapid shallow breathing) and loss of responsiveness.

Heatstroke is a medical emergency. If left untreated, it can cause multiple organ failure, brain damage and death.

Signs and symptoms

- **High body temperature: having a temperature of 40°C (104°F) or above is a major sign of heatstroke**
- **Heavy sweating that suddenly stops: if the body is unable to produce any more sweat then this is a big warning sign that the body has become over-heated and dehydrated**
- **Rapid heartbeat**
- **Rapid breathing**
- **Muscle cramps**

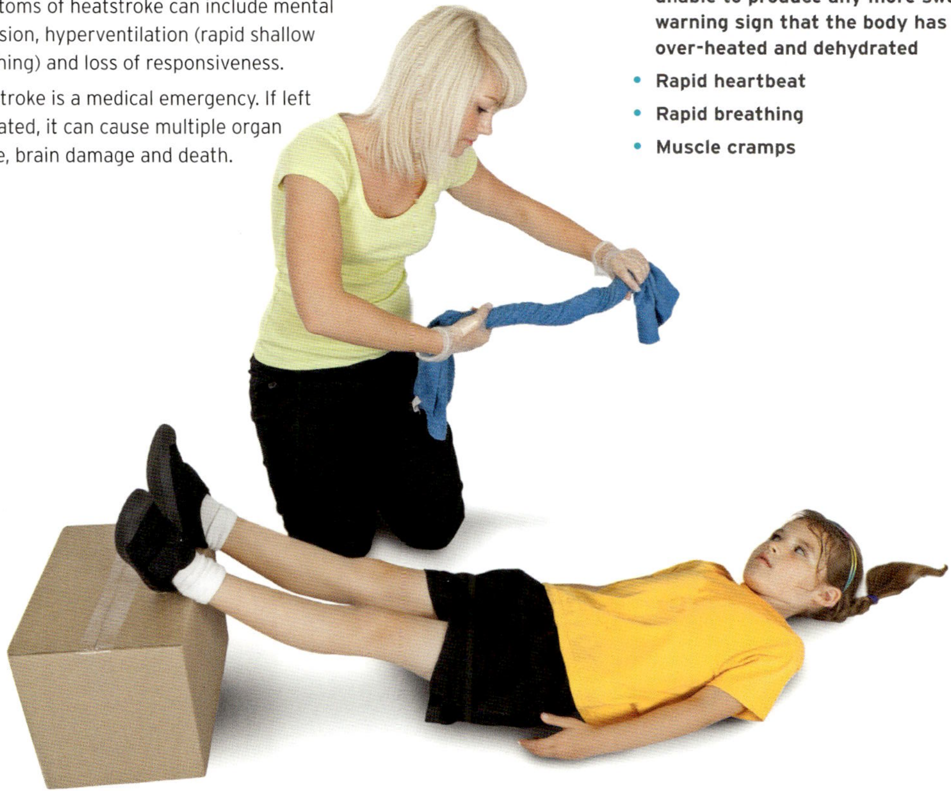

Treatment

- Move the casualty to a cool area as quickly as possible
- Increase the air supply by opening windows or using a fan
- Give them water to drink if possible, but do not give them any medication
- Shower the skin with cool, but not cold, water (15°C-18°C). If there is no shower nearby, cover the body with cool, damp towels or sheets, or immerse in cool water
- Gently massage the skin to encourage circulation
- If seizures start, move nearby objects out of the way to prevent injury (do not use force or put anything in the mouth)
- If the casualty is unresponsive and vomiting, place them in the recovery position
- Call 999/112 for an ambulance

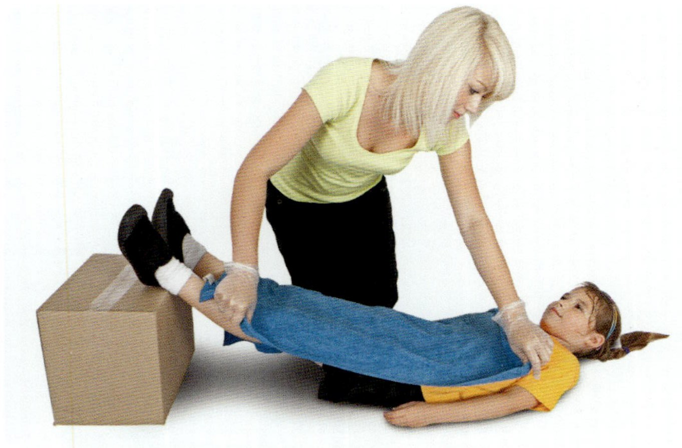

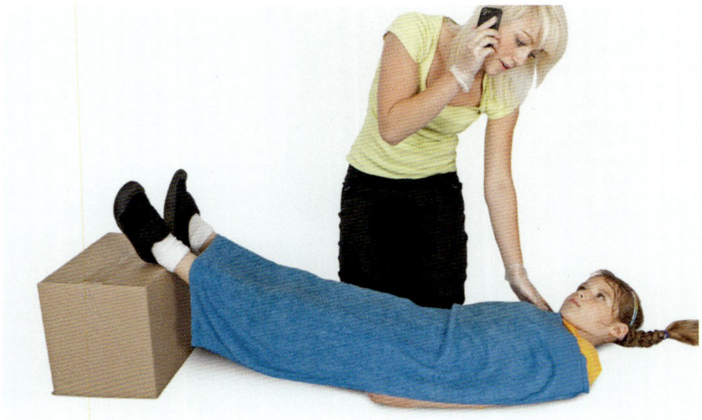

HYPOTHERMIA

Hypothermia occurs when a person's normal body temperature of around 37°C (98.6°F) drops below 35°C (95°F).

It is usually caused by being in a cold environment. It can be triggered by a combination of things, including prolonged exposure to cold (such as staying outdoors in cold conditions or in a poorly heated room for a long time), rain, wind, sweat, inactivity or being in cold water.

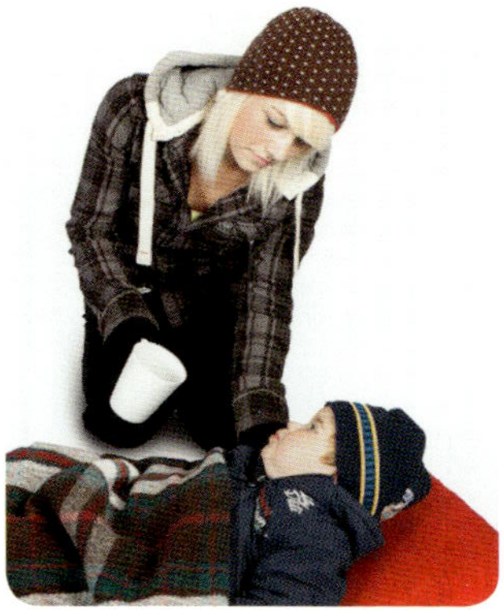

Signs and symptoms

The symptoms of hypothermia depend on how cold the environment is and how long your casualty is exposed for.

Severe hypothermia needs urgent medical treatment in hospital. Shivering is a good guide to how severe the condition is. If the person can stop shivering on their own, the hypothermia is mild, but if they cannot stop shivering, it is moderate to severe.

MILD CASES

In mild cases, symptoms include:

- **Shivering**
- **Feeling cold**
- **Low energy**
- **Cold, pale skin**

MODERATE CASES

The symptoms of moderate hypothermia include:

- **Violent, uncontrollable shivering**
- **Being unable to think or pay attention**
- **Confusion (some people don't realise they are affected)**
- **Loss of judgement and reasoning**
- **Difficulty moving around or stumbling** (weakness)
- **Feeling afraid**
- **Memory loss**
- **Fumbling hands and loss of coordination**
- **Drowsiness**
- **Slurred speech**
- **Listlessness and indifferent**
- **Slow, shallow breathing and a weak pulse**

SEVERE CASES

The symptoms of severe hypothermia include:

- **Loss of control of hands, feet, and limbs**
- **Uncontrollable shivering that suddenly stops**
- **Unresponsiveness**
- **Shallow or no breathing**
- **Weak, irregular or no pulse**
- **Stiff muscles**
- **Dilated pupils**

Treating hypothermia at home

As hypothermia can be a life-threatening condition, seek medical attention as soon as possible.

Hypothermia is treated by preventing further heat being lost and by gently warming the casualty.

If you are treating someone with mild hypothermia at home, or waiting for medical treatment to arrive, follow the advice below to prevent further loss of heat.

- **Move the casualty indoors, or somewhere warm, as soon as possible**
- **Once sheltered, gently remove any wet clothing and dry them**
- **Wrap them in blankets, towels, coats (whatever you have), protecting the head and torso first**
- **Increase activity if possible, but not to the point where sweating occurs, as that cools the skin down again**
- **If possible, give them warm drinks (but not alcohol) or high energy foods, such as chocolate, to help warm them up**
- **Once their body temperature has increased, keep them warm and dry**

It is important to handle anyone that has hypothermia very gently and carefully.

Things you should NOT do:

- **Do not warm up an elderly person using a bath, as this may send cold blood from the body's surfaces to the heart or brain too suddenly, causing a stroke or heart attack**
- **Do not apply direct heat (hot water or a heating pad, for example) to the arms and legs, as this forces cold blood back to the major organs, making the condition worse**
- **Do not give them alcohol to drink, as this will decrease the body's ability to retain heat**
- **Do not rub or massage their skin, as this can cause the blood vessels to widen and decrease the body's ability to retain heat. In severe cases of hypothermia there is also a risk of heart attack**

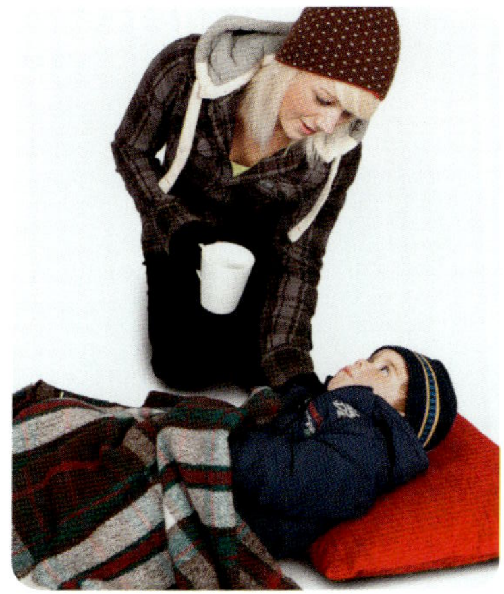

When to seek medical help

If someone you know has been exposed to the cold and they're distressed or confused, and they have slow, shallow breathing or they're unresponsive, they may have severe hypothermia. Their skin may look healthy but feel cold. Babies may also be limp, unusually quiet and refuse to feed.

Cases of severe hypothermia require urgent medical treatment in hospital. You should call 999 to request an ambulance if you suspect that someone you know has severe hypothermia. Do not give them any food or drink.

As the body temperature drops, shivering will stop completely. The heart rate will slow and your casualty will gradually lose responsiveness.

Be prepared to resuscitate if they stop breathing normally.

ELECTRIC SHOCK INCIDENTS

ELECTRICITY

Electrical burns can be caused by lightning or from a man made source involving either, a high-voltage supply e.g. overhead power lines, or from a low-voltage supply as found in the home, or at work.

In all cases, an electrical injury can be life-threatening.

You may have multiple injuries to treat, including cessation of breathing, and a wound that enters the body as well as one that exits the body.

Your first priority is to ensure that it is safe to offer your casualty treatment.

In respect of a high-voltage injury, it is imperative that you and all bystanders stay well away from your casualty. Because the supply can 'arc', you must stay at least 13 metres away from the supply source.

You must call the emergency services immediately, detailing the extent of the incident.

In some cases of low-voltage injuries, the casualty may still have a contact with the supply, and therefore be 'live'. You must break the source of supply immediately before attempting any form of treatment. Switch the supply off from the main fuse-board. Failing that, remove the electrical device from the casualty. You can achieve this by standing on a dry insulating material such as a book or telephone directory. Use a wooden or plastic handle to drag away the source from the casualty ensuring that the area is safe for all.

As soon as you have deemed it safe to do so, you may start your treatment.

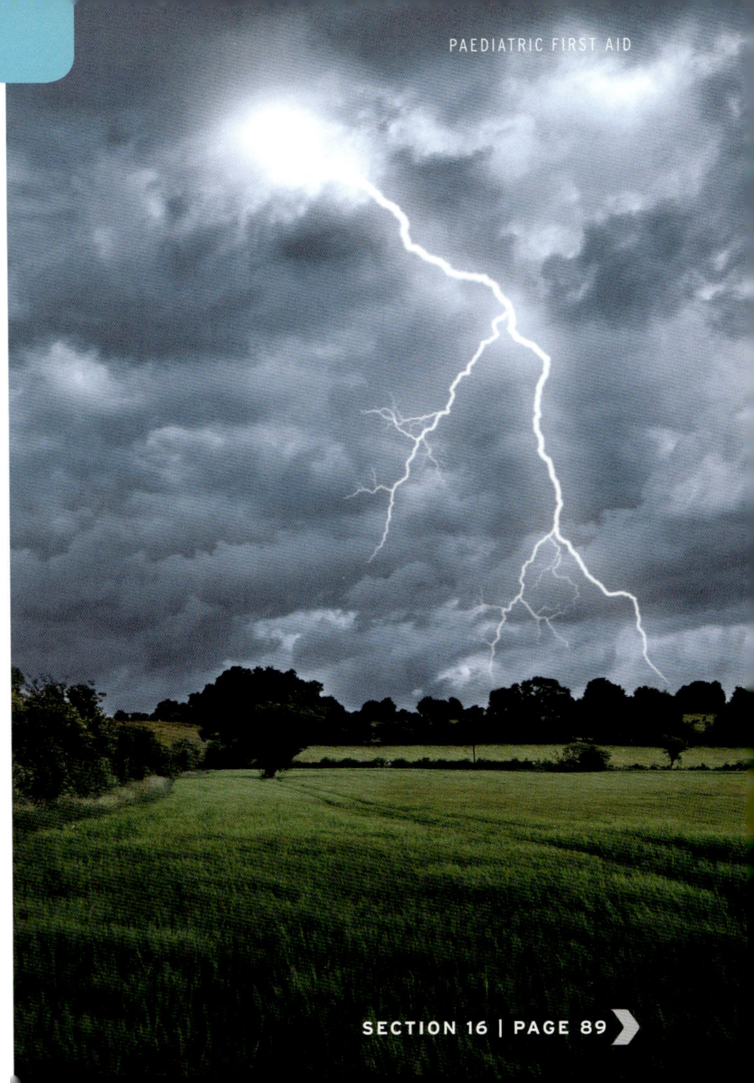

Treatment

LIGHTNING STRIKE

Only when it is safe to do so:

- Carry out your basic life support procedures
- Call for the emergency services
- Be aware of any potential serious burns to deal with

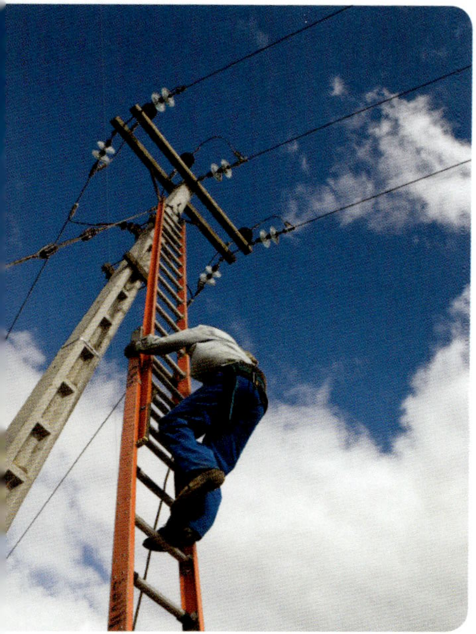

HIGH-VOLTAGE INJURIES

- Keep everyone at least 18 metres away from the electrical source
- Call for the emergency services
- Only when it is safe to do so, as directed by the emergency services, carry out your basic life support procedures

LOW-VOLTAGE INJURIES

- Switch off from the MAINS supply
- Break contact between the electricity and your casualty
- If you are unable to do this, you must insulate yourself before attempting to free your casualty from the supply

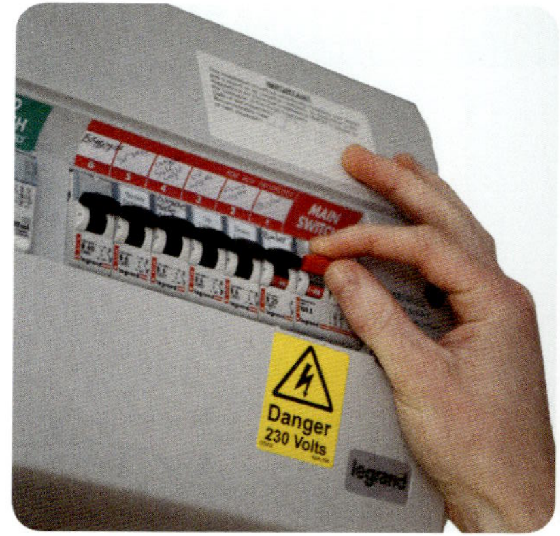

Once your casualty is free from the supply:

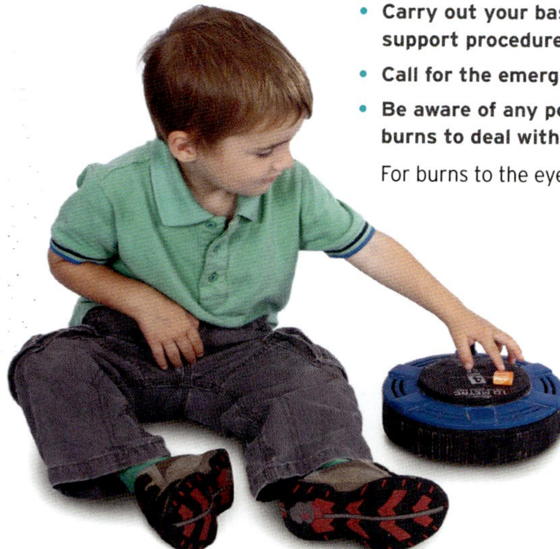

- Carry out your basic life support procedures
- Call for the emergency services
- Be aware of any potential serious burns to deal with

For burns to the eyes (see page 76)

BURNS AND SCALDS

Burns and scalds are among the most serious and painful of injuries. They can be caused by a number of factors including fire, water, electricity, oils, hot surfaces, steam, chemicals and radiation.

CLASSIFICATION OF BURNS

Superficial

The outer layer of skin is burnt causing redness, tenderness and inflammation.

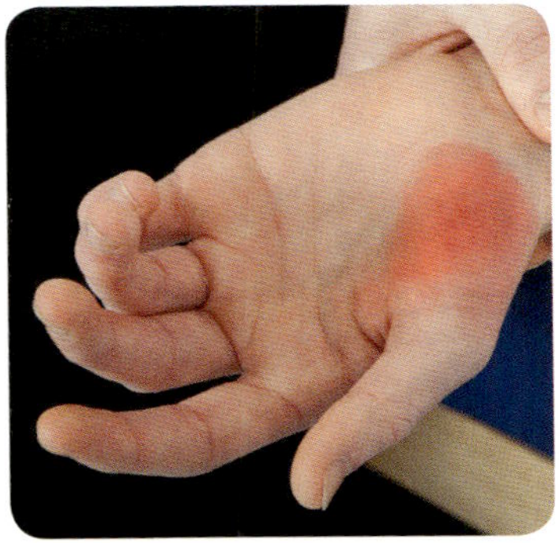

Typical factors causing this would be sunburn or touching a hot iron.

The skin is not broken or blistered.

Partial thickness

The outer layer of the skin is burnt and broken causing blistering, swelling, pain and rawness.

Full thickness

All the layers of skin have been damaged causing the skin to look pale, charred and waxy with fatty deposits. There may also be damage to the nerves.

When to send a casualty to hospital

Every year in the UK, around 175,000 people attend hospital accident and emergency departments for burns injuries.

People who may be at greater risk from the effects of burns, such as children under five years of age and pregnant women, should seek medical attention after a burn or scald.

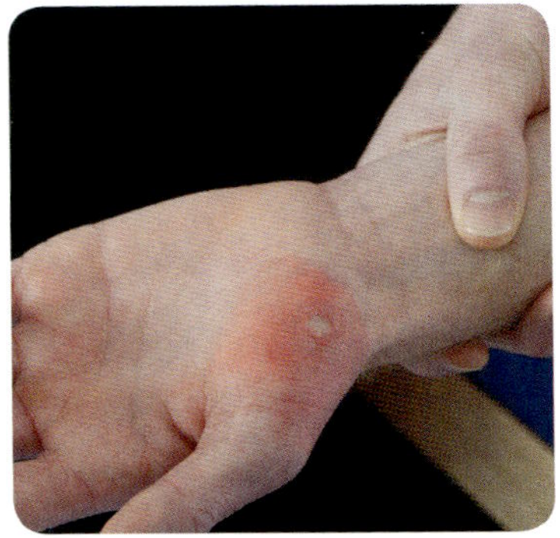

Assessing the extent of the burn

One quick way to estimate the surface area that has been burned is to compare it to the size of the palm of the casualty's hand, which is roughly equal to 1% of the body's total surface area.

For other groups, you must send them to hospital if:

- **The burns affect the hands, feet, face and genital areas**
- **Full thickness burns**
- **Burns that extend around a limb**
- **All partial thickness burns larger than 1% of the body's surface. The casualty's hand represents about 1% on the body's surface**
- **All superficial burns that represent 5% of the body's surface**
- **Burns with a mixed pattern of depth**

If you are in any doubt, then you should seek medical advice.

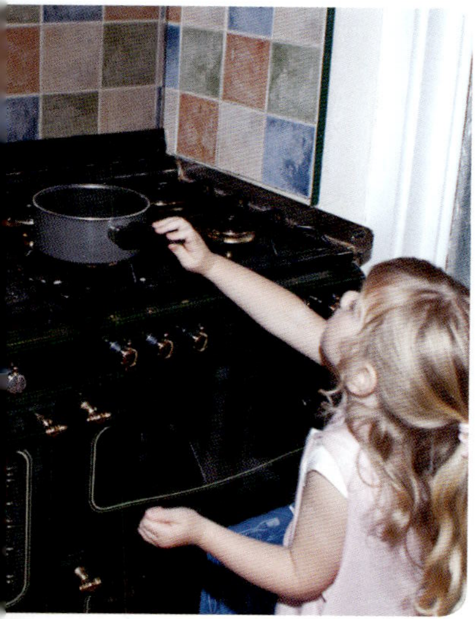

Treatment of burns

- Ensure the area is safe, particularly from the source that created the burn or scald
- Wear disposable gloves
- If it's possible, remove the watch and any jewellery around the affected area
- Cool the burn with cool running tap water for 20 minutes
- Cover the burn with a suitable sterile dressing that is not fluffy. You can cover it with cling film if you have no appropriate dressing
- Treat the casualty for shock
- Monitor their condition throughout and call for an ambulance if it deteriorates
- Remove them to hospital if you consider it appropriate

You must not:

- Apply any form of cream, ointment or fat to the affected area
- Burst any blister that may form
- Apply any form of adhesive dressing
- Remove anything that is stuck to the affected area

NB: The biggest risk associated with bursting blisters is infection

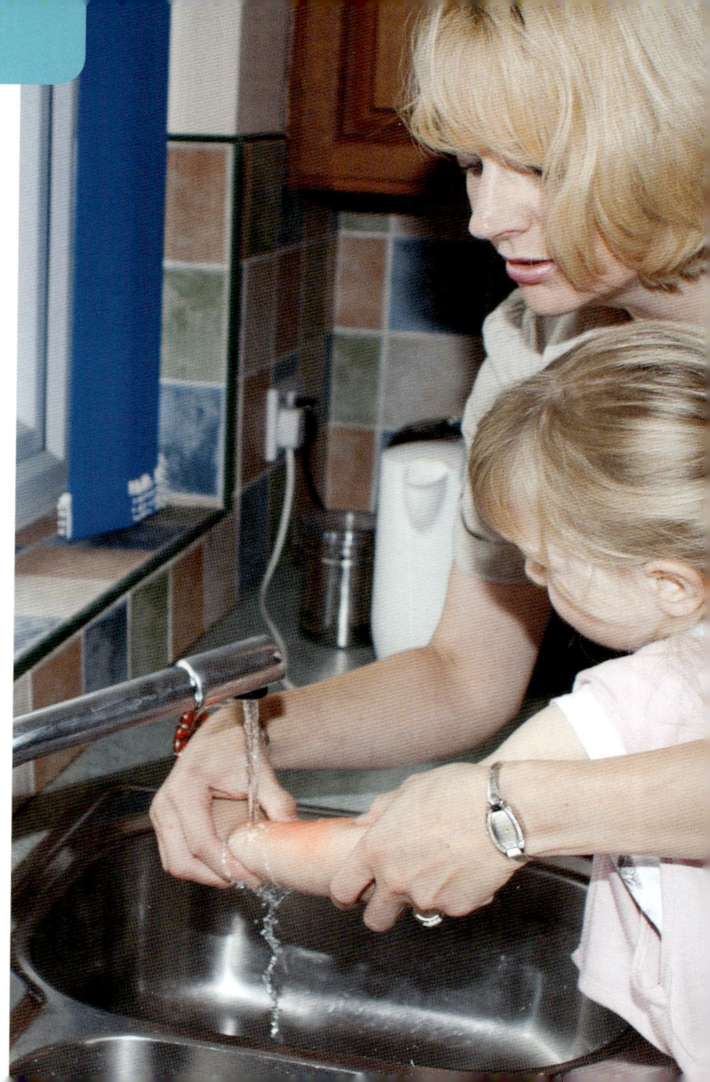

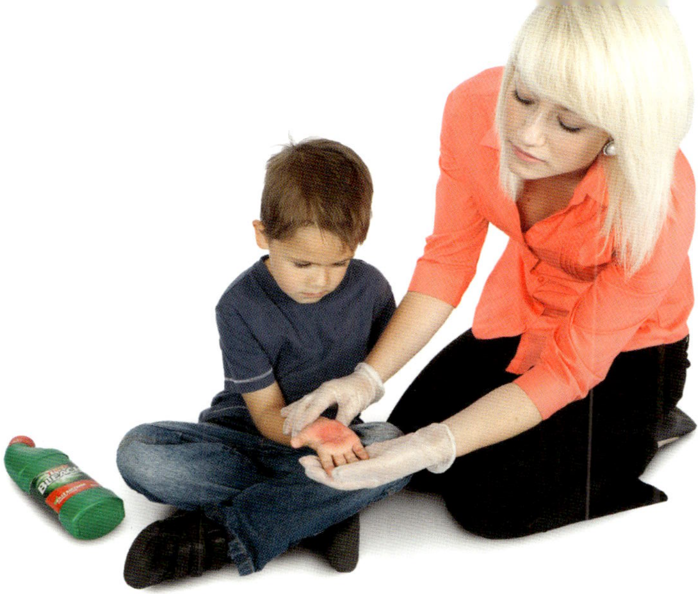

Treating chemical burns

If your casualty is suffering a burn from a chemical, a bleach or acid you should:

- **Remove any chemicals from the skin by running the affected area under cool tap water for 20 minutes, or more. If the chemical involved is in powder form, such as lime, brush it off the skin before running the skin under water**
- **Remove any jewellery or clothing that may have been exposed to the chemical**
- **Apply a cool wet towel to help relieve pain**
- **Cover the burnt skin with a dry sterile dressing, or clean cloth**
- **If your casualty experiences an increased sensation of burning, rewash the skin for a further 10 minutes**
- **Take your casualty to hospital for the extent of the burn to be assessed**

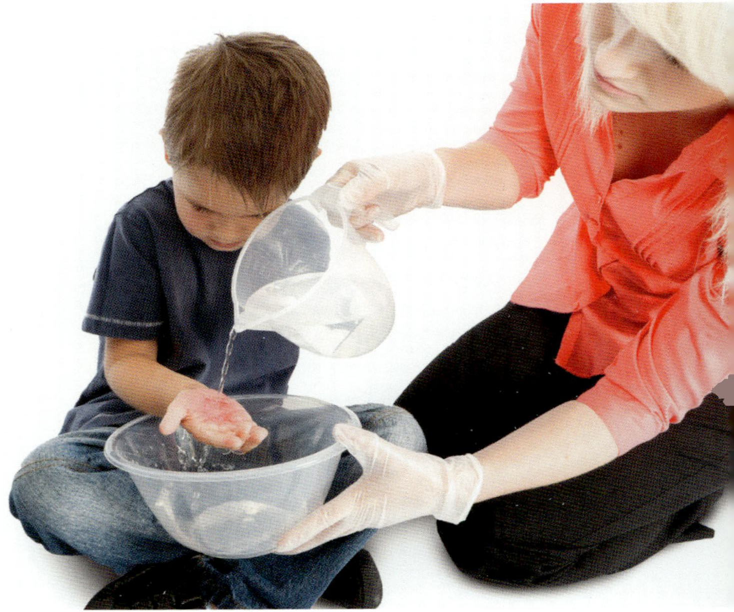

POISONING

Poisoning happens when you take into your body, a substance that damages your cells and organs, and injures your health.

Poisons are usually swallowed, but they can also be inhaled, splashed onto the skin or eyes, injected or received through a bite (as with snake bites).

Many substances are only poisonous if an abnormally large amount is taken. For example, paracetamol is harmless if you take one or two tablets for a headache, but is poisonous if you take an overdose.

A poison can enter the body in a number of ways:

- **Inhaled** Gases, fumes etc
- **Swallowed** Food, alcohol, drugs etc
- **Injected** Drugs, medicine, stings etc
- **Absorbed** Chemicals, vapours etc - through the skin
- **Instilled** Chemicals and gases etc - via the eyes

General treatment for poisons

- **Call for an ambulance immediately**
- **Place in the recovery position in order to maintain an open airway, and to allow vomit to drain from the mouth**
- **Keep any evidence of the poison**
- **Monitor their breathing and be prepared to resuscitate them**

HOUSEHOLD POISONS

Bleach, oven cleaner, paint stripper etc

Recognition if it is swallowed

- **Redness, blistering, burns and swelling to the face, mouth and lips**
- **Distressed breathing, leading to unresponsiveness**

Treatment

- **Check the airway and their breathing. Be prepared to resuscitate** (use a face shield)
- **Call for an ambulance**
- **If the casualty is responsive, keep them sat up and give them sips of water to dilute. Identify the poison that was taken**
- **Do not induce vomiting**

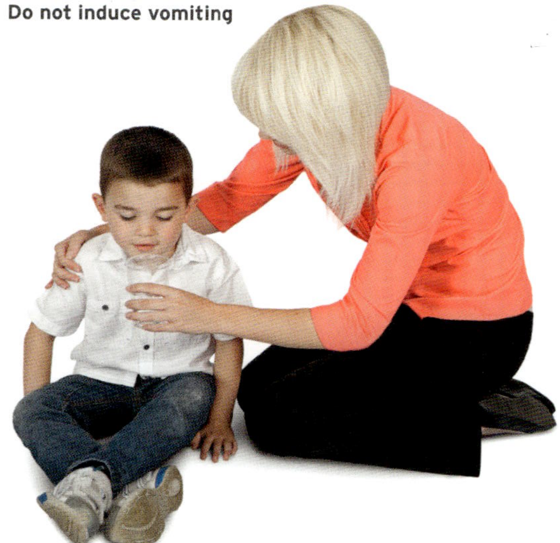

INDUSTRIAL POISONS

Corrosive chemicals and gases

Recognition

- Possible burning sensation in the airway and skin
- Breathing difficulties
- Burns around the body
- Possible coughing and sneezing
- Nausea and vomiting
- Severe headache and disorientation
- Unresponsiveness

Treatment

- Call for an ambulance immediately
- Protect yourself
- Remove the casualty from the source
- Move them into fresh air
- Treat the appropriate condition such as a burn
- If they become unresponsive, place them in the recovery position and monitor their breathing
- Be prepared to resuscitate them

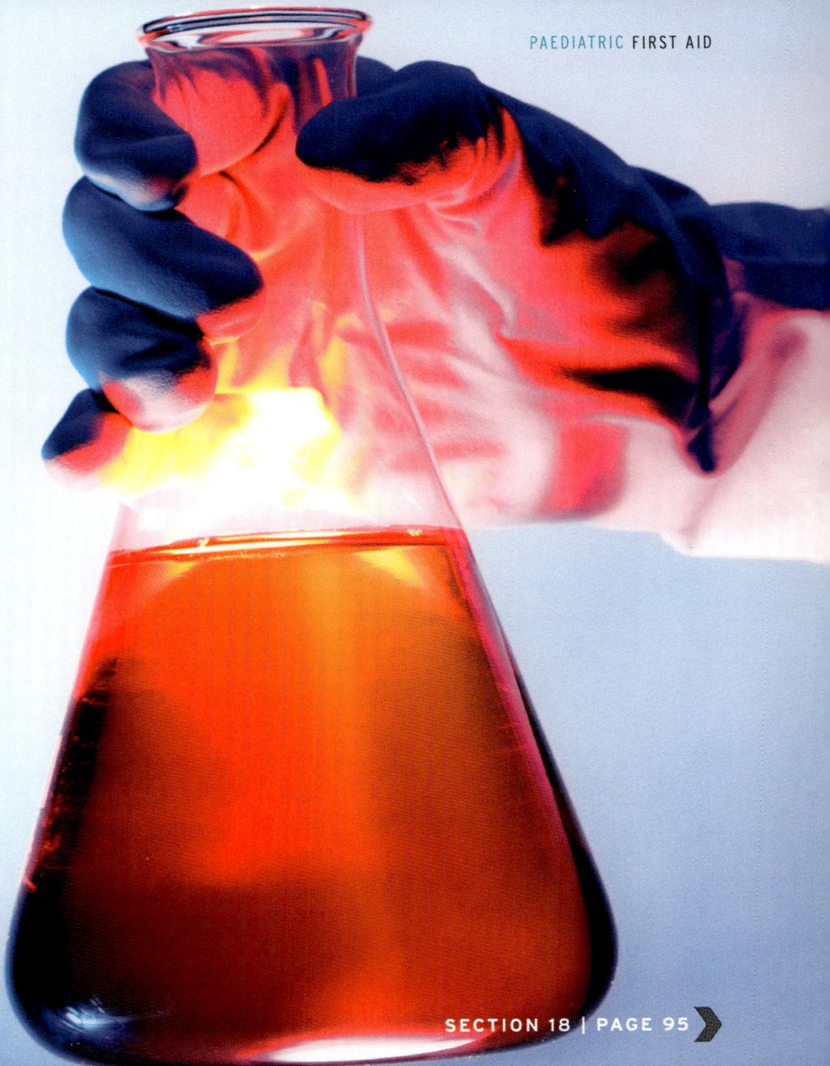

DRUG POISONING OR OVERDOSE

Recognition

ASPIRIN

- Upper abdominal pain
- Nausea and vomiting
- Ringing in the ears
- Confusion and delirium
- 'Sighing' when breathing
- Dizziness

PARACETAMOL

- Developing abdominal pains
- Nausea and vomiting

TRANQUILLISERS (ANTI-DEPRESSANTS)

- Lethargy, sleepiness leading to unresponsiveness
- Shallow breathing
- Weak, irregular pulse

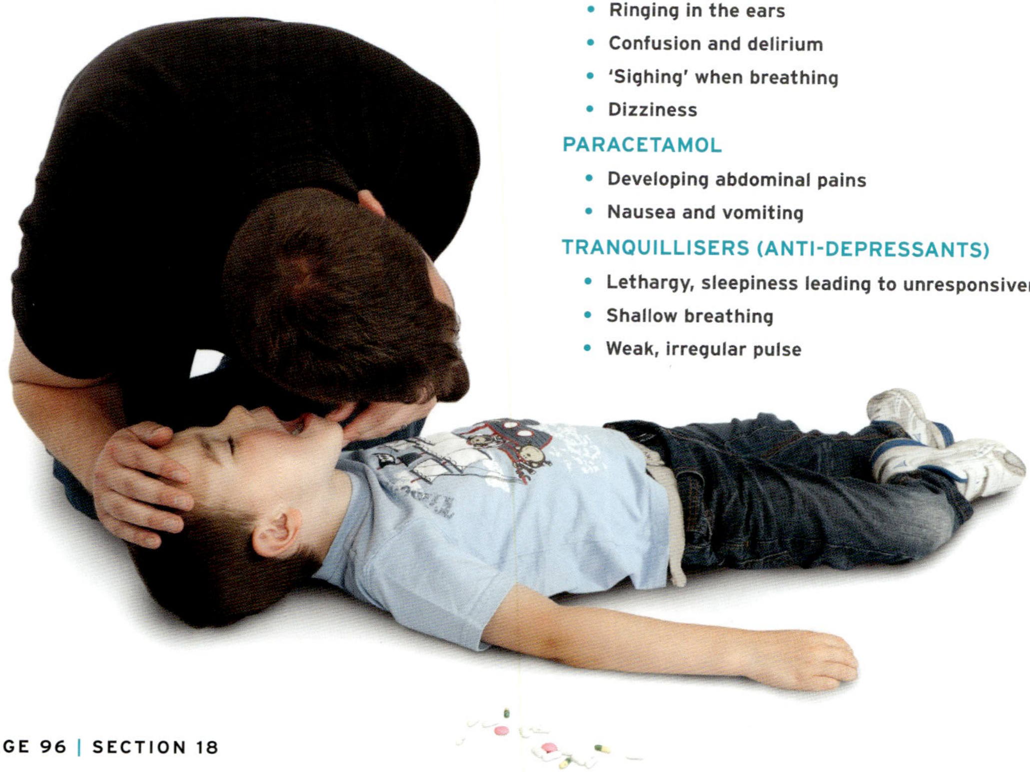

NARCOTICS

- Small pupils
- Sluggishness and confusion, possibly leading to unresponsiveness
- Slow, shallow breathing which may stop
- Needle marks which may be infected

SOLVENTS

- Nausea and vomiting
- Headaches
- Hallucinations
- Unresponsiveness - possibly

STIMULANTS

- Excitable, hyperactive behaviour, wildness and frenzy
- Sweating
- Tremors
- Hallucinations

Treatment

- Protect yourself
- If responsive, place them in a comfortable position and try to establish the drug that has been taken
- Call for an ambulance
- Monitor their breathing
- Keep samples of vomited material and try to find evidence of the drug that was taken
- Be prepared to resuscitate

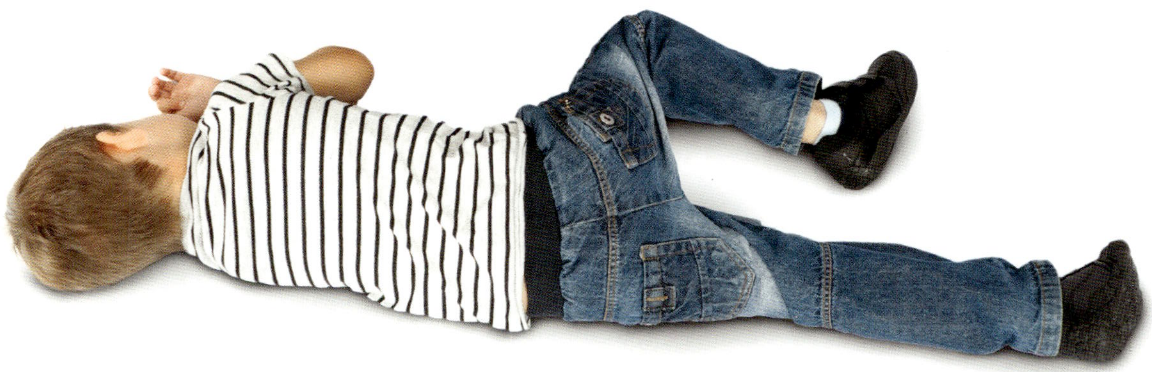

POISONING continued

PLANT POISONING

Most plants that grow in the UK are harmless and, if eaten, may only cause a mild stomach upset.

Some types of plant can have a more serious effect, so it is important to know what plants are growing in your garden.

If a potentially poisonous plant has been eaten, try to identify it so you can inform medical staff, or take a sample with you to the hospital so that it can be identified.

The plants to look out for include, Wild Arum, Foxglove, Laburnum, Death Cap mushrooms, Ivy and Mistletoe - to name a few.

Recognition

- **Nausea and vomiting**
- **Abdominal pains**
- **Diarrhoea**
- **Seizures**
- **Impaired responsiveness**

Treatment

The same treatment can be applied as you would for drug poisoning (see page 84).

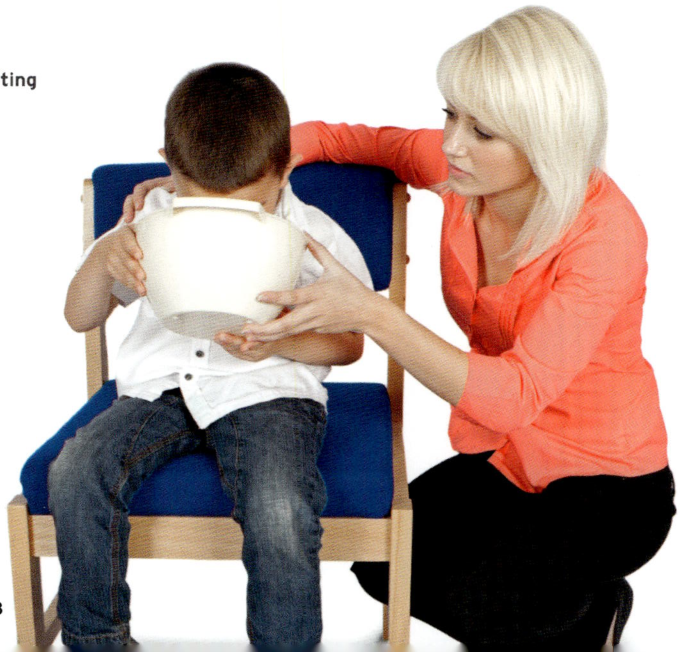

FOOD POISONING

This is usually caused by consuming contaminated food or drink. Some food poisoning is caused by foods that already have the bacteria in it, particularly from the E.Coli or salmonella group of bacteria.

This particular poison could take hours or days before it takes effect.

The other main group are poisons produced by staphylococcus. The symptoms of poisoning develop far more rapidly, normally within 2-6 hours.

Recognition

- **Nausea and vomiting**
- **Abdominal pains**
- **Diarrhoea**
- **Fever**
- **Headache**
- **Impaired responsiveness**

Treatment

- **Encourage the casualty to rest**
- **Offer them plenty of bland fluids to drink**
- **Try to establish the source of the poisoning in case medical assistance is required**
- **Call for an ambulance if their condition deteriorates**

ALCOHOL POISONING

Alcohol poisoning results from drinking a toxic amount of alcohol, usually over a short period of time, which is known as binge drinking.

On rare occasions, alcohol poisoning can occur if you accidentally drink household products that contain alcohol.

The intake of alcohol depresses the activity of the central nervous system, particularly the brain. Prolonged or excessive intake can severely impair all physical and mental functions and the casualty may become unresponsive.

Recognition

- **Smell of alcohol**
- **Evidence of empty containers**
- **Impaired unresponsiveness, leading to unresponsiveness**
- **Flushed appearance**
- **Deep, noisy breathing**

In the later stages of unresponsiveness:

- **Dry, bloated appearance to the face**
- **Shallow breathing**
- **Weak and rapid pulse**
- **Dilated pupils**

Treatment

- **Place them in the recovery position to maintain an open airway**
- **Monitor their breathing**
- **Keep them warm**
- **Seek medical assistance if there is another condition, such as a head injury to deal with**

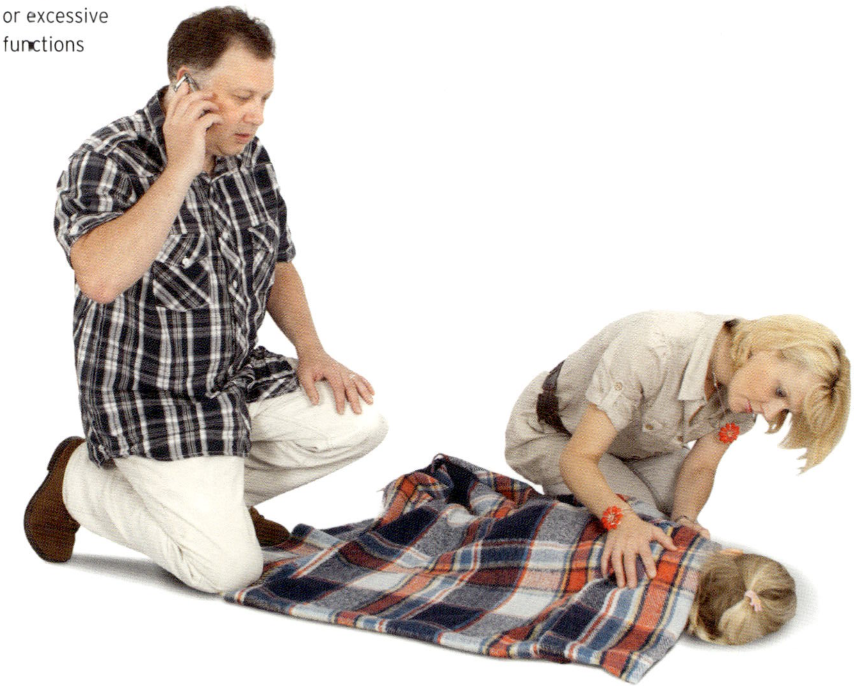

ANAPHYLAXIS

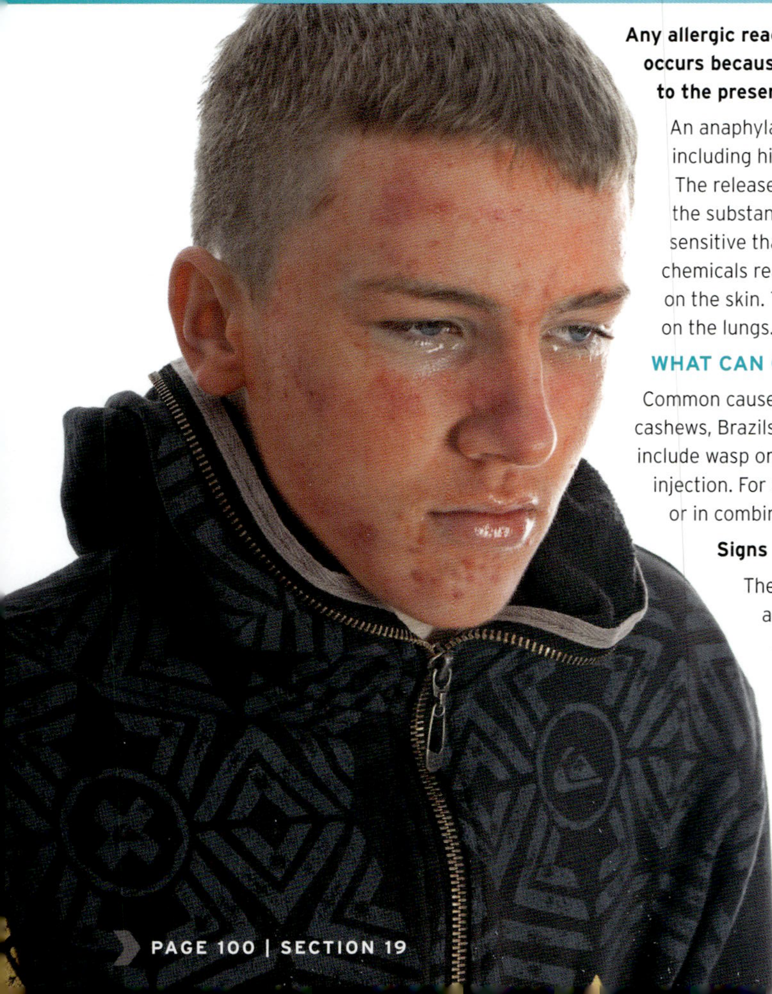

Any allergic reaction including the most extreme form, anaphylactic shock, occurs because the body's immune system reacts inappropriately in response to the presence of a substance that it wrongly perceives as a threat.

An anaphylactic reaction is caused by the sudden release of chemical substances, including histamine, from cells in the blood and tissues where they are stored. The release is triggered by the reaction between the allergic antibody (IgE) and the substance (allergen) causing the anaphylactic reaction. This mechanism is so sensitive that minute quantities of the allergen can cause a reaction. The released chemicals react on blood vessels to cause the swelling in the mouth and anywhere on the skin. There is a fall in blood pressure and, in asthmatics; the effect is mainly on the lungs.

WHAT CAN CAUSE ANAPHYLAXIS?

Common causes include foods such as peanuts, tree nuts (e.g. almonds, walnuts, cashews, Brazils), sesame, fish, shellfish, dairy products and eggs. Non-food causes include wasp or bee stings, natural latex (rubber), penicillin or any other drug or injection. For some people, exercise can trigger a severe reaction - either on its own or in combination with other factors such as food or drugs (e.g. aspirin).

Signs and symptoms

The symptoms of anaphylaxis usually start between 3 and 60 minutes after contact with the allergen. Less commonly, they can occur a few hours or even days after contact.

When your casualty has an anaphylactic reaction, they may feel unwell or dizzy or may faint because of a sudden drop in blood pressure.

Narrowing of the airways can also occur at the same time, with or without the drop in blood pressure. This can cause breathing difficulties and wheezing.

Your casualty may also experience any of the symptoms below:

- **Swollen eyes, lips, hands, feet and other areas**
- **A strange metallic taste in the mouth**
- **Sore, red, itchy eyes**
- **Changes in heart rate**
- **A sudden feeling of extreme anxiety or apprehension**
- **Itchy skin or nettle-rash** (hives)
- **Unresponsiveness due to very low blood pressure**
- **Abdominal cramps, vomiting or diarrhoea**
- **Nausea and fever**

Your casualty would not necessarily experience all of these symptoms.

Adrenaline is the gold standard in the treatment of anaphylaxis, and its administration should not be delayed.

In a First Aid situation, adrenalin will normally be delivered by an auto-injector.

If available, an injection of adrenaline should be given as soon as possible.

If after 5 - 15 minutes the casualty still feels unwell, a second injection should be given. This should be given in the opposite thigh.

A second dose may also be required if the symptoms reoccur.

When treating a potential anaphylaxis casualty, it should be noted that there are **NO** contraindications for the use of adrenaline.

Treatment for a severe reaction

- **Call for an ambulance immediately**
- **If your casualty is having difficulty breathing, help them to sit up**
- **If they have low blood pressure, get them to lie flat and raise their legs**
- **If they are unresponsive, check that their airway is open and clear, and check that they are breathing normally**
- **Place them in the recovery position**
- **Be prepared to resuscitate**

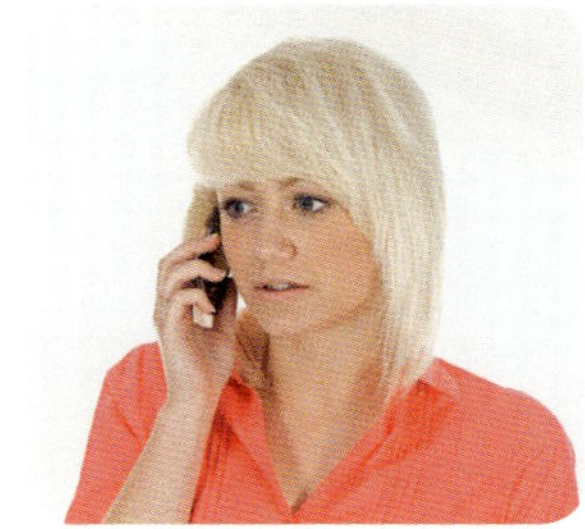

What the HSE say:

Medicines legislation restricts the administration of injectable medicines.

Unless self-administered, they may only be administered by, or in accordance with, the instructions of a doctor (e.g. by a nurse).

However, in the case of adrenaline there is an exemption to this restriction, which means in an emergency a layperson is permitted to administer it by injection for the purpose of saving life.

When can an Epipen be used?

The use of an Epipen to treat anaphylactic shock is an example of an exemption from the restriction imposed by medicines legislation.

Therefore, First Aiders may administer an Epipen if they are dealing with a life-threatening emergency involving a casualty who has been prescribed and is in possession of an Epipen, and where the First Aider is trained to use it.

ADULT BASIC LIFE SUPPORT

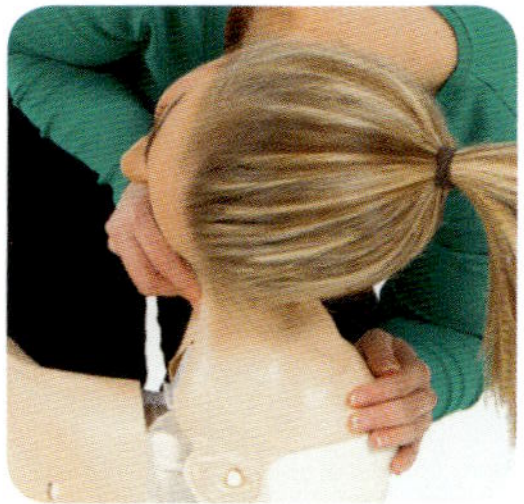

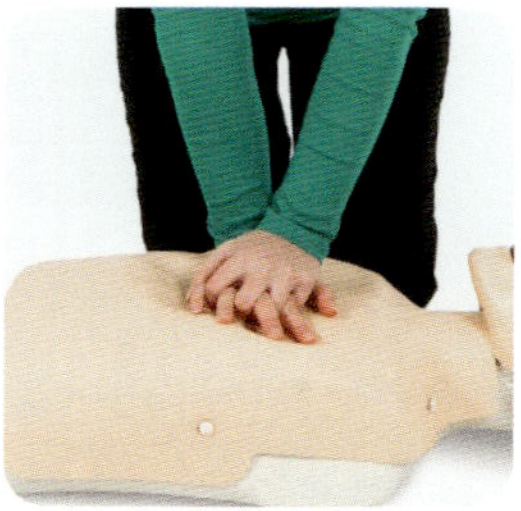

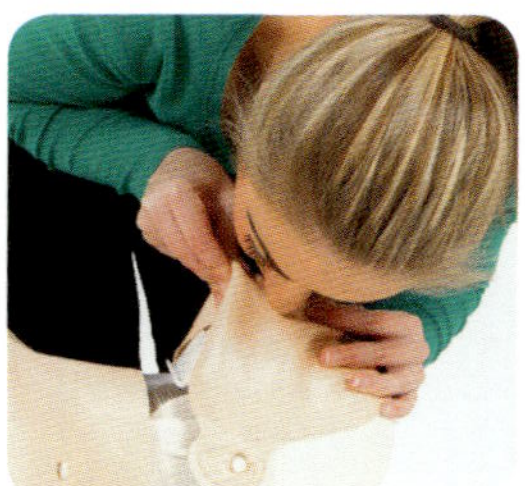

CHECK FOR DANGERS

CHECK FOR RESPONSE

- **YES** → If responsive, check for injuries and treat accordingly. Call the emergency services if required.
- **NO** → If you are on your own, you should shout for help. Ideally you should never leave your casualty on their own.

OPEN THE AIRWAY → Use minimum head tilt and lift the chin carefully.

Check for normal breathing for no more than 10 seconds.

- **YES** → If breathing normally, check for any injuries and place them in the recovery position. Call the emergency services and monitor their breathing.
- **NO** ↓

If help is available, send them to call the emergency services and to bring a defibrillator back with them if one is available.

- **NO** → If no help is available you must call them yourself and return with a defibrillator if one is available. (then → Give 30 chest compressions followed by 2 breaths.)
- **YES** ↓

Give 30 chest compressions followed by 2 breaths.

Continue with CPR until the casualty recovers, the emergency services take over or you become exhausted.

NB: If a defibrillator is available, then connect it immediately to the casualty and follow the voice prompts. If you have trained help available, then they can start CPR whilst you are preparing the casualty for defibrillation. (If you have access to an AED - See pages 25-29)

ADULT RESUSCITATION

1. Start with 30 chest compressions

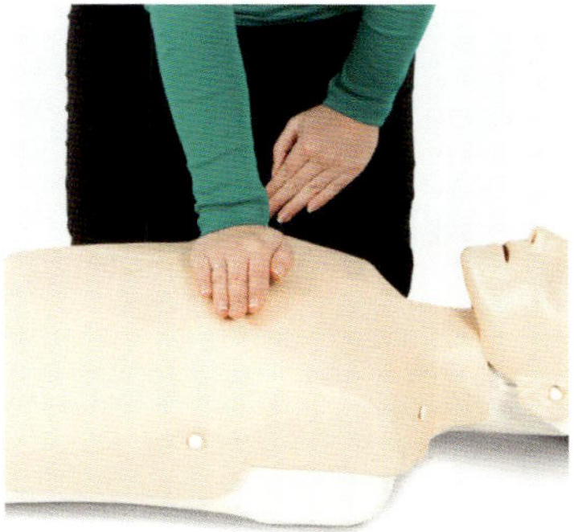

- **Kneel by the side of your casualty**
- **Place the heel of one hand in the centre of the casualty's chest** (which is the lower half of the casualty's breastbone (sternum)

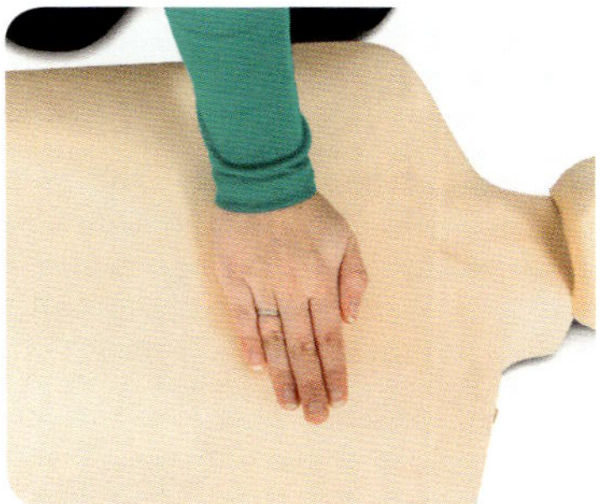

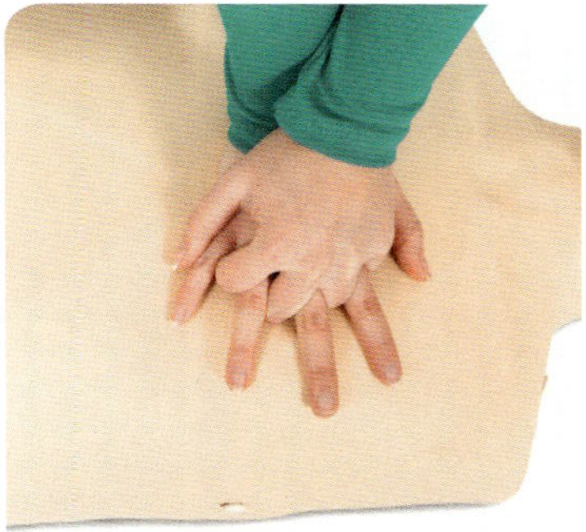

- **Place the heel of your other hand on top of the first hand**
- **Interlock the fingers of your hands and ensure that pressure is not applied over their ribs. Do not apply any pressure over the upper abdomen or the bottom end of the sternum**
- **Position yourself vertically above their chest and, with your arms straight, press down on the sternum approximately 5cm (But not more than 6cm)**

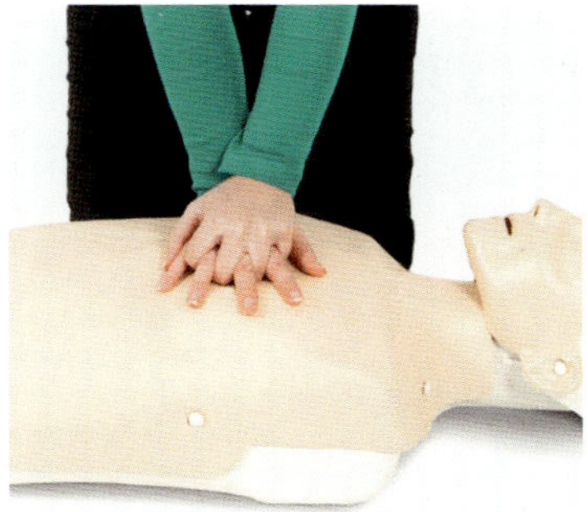

- **After each compression, release all the pressure on the chest without losing contact between your hands and the sternum.**
  Do not lean on the chest.
- **Repeat 30 chest compressions at a speed of 100 - 120 compressions per minute with as few interruptions as possible**
- **Compression and release should take an equal amount of time**

In most circumstances it will be possible to identify the correct hand position for chest compressions, without removing the casualty's clothes. If you are in any doubt, then remove outer clothing.

2. Give 2 rescue breaths After 30 chest compressions open the airway again using head tilt and chin lift.

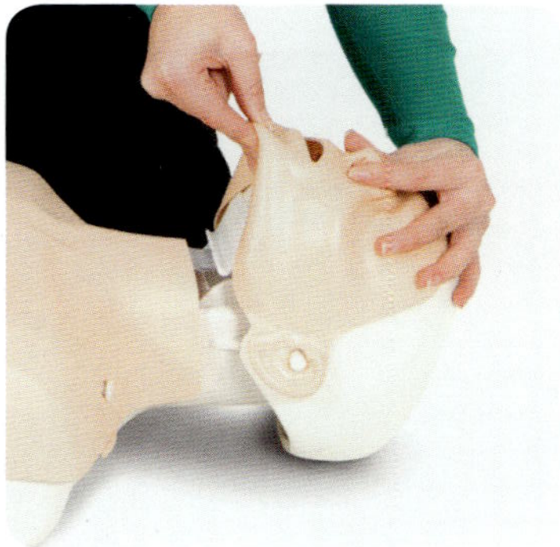

- **Pinch the soft part of their nose closed, using the index finger and thumb of your hand on their forehead**
- **Allow their mouth to open, but maintain chin lift**
- **Take a normal breath and place your lips around their mouth, making sure that you have a good seal**
- **Blow steadily into their mouth whilst watching for their chest to rise, taking about one second as in normal breathing; this is an effective rescue breath**

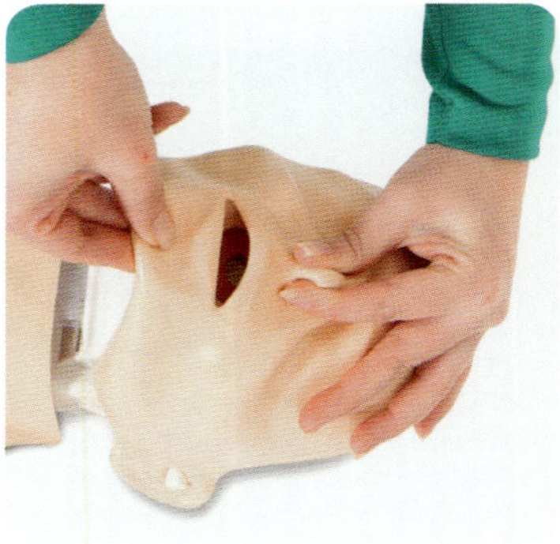

- **Maintaining head tilt and chin lift, watch for their chest to fall as air comes out**
- **Take another normal breath and blow into the casualty's mouth once more to achieve a total of two effective rescue breaths. Do not interrupt compressions by more than 10 seconds to deliver two breaths. Then return your hands without delay to the correct position on the sternum and give a further 30 chest compressions**

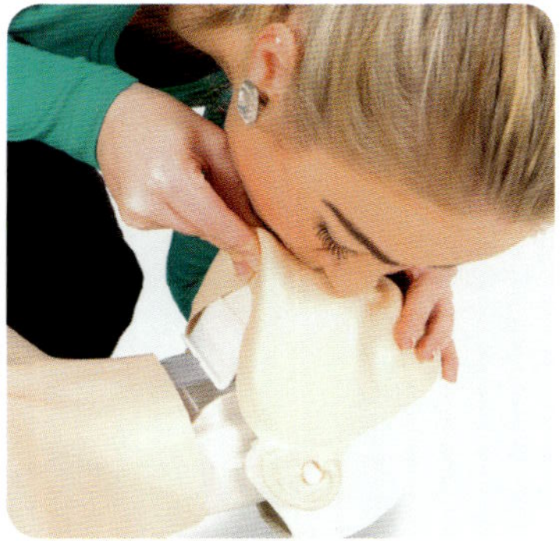

If the initial rescue breath of each sequence does not make the chest rise as in normal breathing, then, before your next attempt:

- **Check the casualty's mouth and remove any visible obstruction**
- **Re-check that there is adequate head tilt and chin lift**
- **Do not attempt more than two breaths each time before returning to chest compressions**